Chasing Zebras

Also by Margaret Nowaczyk

Polish(ed): Poland Rooted in Canadian Fiction (co-edited with Kasia Jaronczyk)
Searching for Ancestors (in Polish)
Your Family Tree of Health (in Polish)

Chasing Zebras

A Memoir of Genetics, Mental Health and Writing

Margaret Nowaczyk

James Street North Books

Published by James Street North Books
an imprint of Wolsak and Wynn Publishers
280 James Street North
Hamilton, ON L8R2L3
www.wolsakandwynn.ca

Editor: Noelle Allen | Copy editor: Andrew Wilmot
Cover and interior design: Rami Schandall/Visual Creative
Cover image: Rami Schandall
Author photograph: Melanie Gordon Photography
Typeset in Freight Text
Printed by Brant Service Press Ltd., Brantford, Canada

Printed on certified 100% post-consumer Rolland Enviro Paper.

10 9 8 7 6 5 4 3 2 1

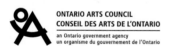 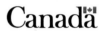

ONTARIO ARTS COUNCIL
CONSEIL DES ARTS DE L'ONTARIO
an Ontario government agency
un organisme du gouvernement de l'Ontario

Canada Council   Conseil des arts
for the Arts   du Canada

Canada

The publisher gratefully acknowledges the support of the Ontario Arts Council, the Canada Council for the Arts and the Government of Canada.

Library and Archives Canada Cataloguing in Publication

Title: Chasing zebras : a memoir of genetics, mental health and writing / Margaret Nowaczyk.
Names: Nowaczyk, Małgorzata (Małgorzata J. M.), author.
Description: Includes bibliographical references.
Identifiers: Canadiana 20210270349 | ISBN 9781989496411 (softcover)
Subjects: LCSH: Nowaczyk, Małgorzata (Małgorzata J. M.) | LCSH: Pediatricians—Canada—Biography. | LCSH: Geneticists—Canada—Biography. | LCSH: Mentally ill—Canada—Biography. | LCSH: Narrative medicine. | CSH: Polish Canadians—Biography. | LCGFT: Autobiographies.
Classification: LCC RJ43.N69 A3 2021 | DDC 618.9200092—dc23

To my teachers and to my patients who also are my teachers

What one has to tell is not nearly so important as the telling itself.

– Henry Miller, "Reflections on Writing," *The Wisdom of the Heart*

When you hear hoofbeats, think horses not zebras.

– Medical school adage

Beginning

"Who wants to read first?" Rita Charon asks our group. A professor of internal medicine and a Henry James scholar, for years she was known at the Columbia medical school as the "crazy book lady" who told anybody who would listen about how reading literature enhanced the practice of medicine.

I have to read. I just have to. I did not travel all the way to New York City to sit this out. This story has been eating at me for almost ten years. I remember the response from a female classmate three years ago when I read what I had written in my first creative writing class: "I hate this. I hate you for making me hear it."

I so hope it will be different here – these are doctors, nurses, social workers who came from around the world to learn how to improve clinical medicine. An inner-city hospital chaplain sits directly across the table from me. They all have witnessed the enduring misery of the human condition, in patients and in doctors. And I want somebody, anybody, to see what my job is about. To see *me*.

I'm attending a narrative medicine workshop at Columbia University Vagelos College of Physicians and Surgeons. In my workshop group are eight health-care professionals, huddled around tables arranged in a circle in a classroom on a glorious October Saturday in New York City. Outside, the leaves on the lindens lining Broadway are beginning to change, and the afternoon sun angles through the tall windows. Narrative medicine, a revolutionary approach to medical care, centres on a patient's story as opposed to their condition, and was conceived and developed at Columbia by Rita Charon. Rita advocated for the study of narrative texts, both literary and spoken, to refine medical history-taking. In addition to the close reading of literary texts to improve a physician's grasp of a patient's medical history, she also uses writing prompts, reflective writing and sharing one's writing with others to support physicians in identifying factors that might be affecting their patient-doctor interactions and deterring them from fully understanding their patients' health stories. As well, these techniques can help physicians process their own emotions. Because as long as a story remains untold and unheard, it festers.

I am about to realize how much.

"Me." I almost shoot my hand up, as I used to in school. It's been a decade and I've never told anybody how I felt. I am hurt, I am upset; I have to share. I must. I don't care if there are others whose need is as great, they will soon see how important, how damaging my story is. I just need to, have to, go first.

My heart pounds so much it hurts. Yes, I know, heartbeat doesn't hurt; what I feel is the increased heart rate and the adrenaline flooding my arteries and veins, the anxiety of unmasking myself and the fear of judgment and rejection on moral grounds. I don't care what the physiological explanation is – my heartbeat hurts.

I read.

When I finish, my cheeks and neck are burning. Already there seems to be more space in my rib cage, in that stiff membrane that has constricted my heart. I glance around. I met these people only the night before, when we shared an innocent icebreaker of a writing prompt: "Tell me the story of your name." What do they think of me now? What I have just read is not the same as "I changed my name from the Polish 'Małgorzata' when a teacher butchered it one time too many." They'd laughed at that. Now, silence pounds in my ears. Are they repulsed by my true colours? Too shocked to even say anything? Angry?

But the faces are not turning away in disgust or recoiling in horror. Nadia, across the table, smiles a kind smile that lights up her face and nods at me.

"What did you hear?" Rita asks.

"How much she's hurting," Thomas says. "How it's eating away at her."

"It's so dark, though," Nadia says.

"How can she make it better for herself?" Rita asks after a pause during which all I hear is my pounding heartbeat.

"She can't change the memory," Krisann says, "but she can change how she looks at it."

"What if ..." Rita stops, thinks. "The name – Savannah. Is that her real name?"

"Yes," I say.

"How about instead of thinking of her being trapped in her body you play with the image of her name – big spaces, the openness of the African savannah. Free, boundless." She peers at me sideways, head tilted like a curious bird. "Hmmm?"

I nod, even though I am not convinced that this mind trick will change anything. I have always thought of Savannah as a ruined medieval castle. But something has already shifted inside me ...

Rita knows what she's talking about.

"It feels so ... so great to have read it," I blurt out. My voice is shaking. "It makes such a difference that you all listened."

Rita watches me seriously. Waits.

"See?" she says finally, her warm grey eyes on me. "You made room for more."

❦

That day, narrative medicine crowbarred open the locked chambers of my heart and mind – the places where I stored my shame and pain. The loneliness of my first years in Canada. The sick competitiveness of my pre-med years. The shocks of medical school and residency. The crazy temper and mood swings that left me with no friends. Bearing witness to the savage heartbreaks of prenatal diagnosis and predictive genetic testing. Lifelong troubles with mental health issues – years of therapy, medications, psychiatrists, psychologists, hospitalization. Crawling back to a normal life.

Since then, words had poured out of me and onto the page, blue on yellow foolscap – my favourite writing medium. My words freed up space in my mind and body, making room for understanding and acceptance, but I needed more than writing out what lurks in the dark recesses of my heart. Sharing and acceptance turned out to be my greatest medicine. Like lancing a boil, the hurt and pain had poured out of me, and my spirit had, finally, begun to heal.

My experiences, many of them traumatic, lived – ineffably, wordlessly – inside me for many years; there, they did a lot of damage. Only when I allowed them out was I able to see who I might be without them – in writing, we make our minds visible to ourselves and others.

Writing, I healed. I moved from being stuck in awfulness to becoming more able and adaptable, even if committing to a version of events that can't easily be "taken back" was scary as hell. But I wanted to tell my story because I wanted it to enable others to tell theirs.

Writing allows our experiences to become universal – through it, we move away from the conviction that they are ours and ours alone. Having written and shared our writing, we emerge from isolation. Listeners – readers – are necessary for the work to be seen, heard, validated and, hopefully, reflected back to us so that we can see what we still have to learn.

Part One

Signs & Symptoms

1

The day the University of Toronto Faculty of Medicine letter of acceptance arrived, I was preparing an agarose gel to separate human saliva proteins in the Bennick lab. My mother phoned the professor's office and read the letter to me. "I did it!" I shouted. Or maybe I just pumped my fist and squealed, "Yessssss!"

July 18, 1985, was no different than any other day that summer: hot, humid, hazy. I stood on the crumbling top stair of the Medical Sciences Building's terrace and scanned the university's Front Campus. The sandstone University College buildings loomed across the verdant lawn and the scent of the camomile trodden by Frisbee throwers wafted toward me; the neo-Gothic Sigmund Samuel Library and the 1960s Science and Medicine Library were to my right. The University Bookroom, where, in the basement, I had been sneaking peeks at medical textbooks for three years, stood tucked in the corner diagonally across from me and Convocation Hall, with its green dome topped with a flagpole, lay to my left. Students and assorted adults – faculty, staff and a clutch of tourists pointing their cameras every which way – went on about their lives. Leashed dogs peed on the trunks of acacia trees circling the lawn. Somehow, inexplicably, life went on. No parades, no marching bands. How could the world be the same if I had just gotten into medical school?

An ambulance siren wailed from the direction of University Avenue, its sound Dopplering as it sped toward one of the downtown hospitals and I thought, a bit melodramatically, "Soon, I'll be at the other end of that ambulance ride." Without any outward signs, life *had* changed. It was going to be so easy from now on: I would finish med school, become a doctor; I would be respected and I would always have a job. It would be a well-paying and prestigious job in a field that had captivated me since before I could read, sneaking peeks at the pages of the Polish *Little Encyclopedia of Health* that I wasn't allowed to touch. As family lore tells it, though I don't remember it, I first announced that I wanted to be a doctor when I was five years old. And despite brief detours of wanting to become an architect, a chemist, a biochemist and – quite out of character – an English professor, that desire held true throughout my life. I never thought the job would be difficult; I was simply fascinated with how the human body was put together and how it worked.

Did I mention that I had just been accepted into medical school?

☞

I had arrived in Toronto only four years earlier with my parents and six-year-old sister, Monika. I was sixteen years old. That first day in Toronto – March 3, 1981 – was cold and dreary; the kind of afternoon I would soon learn typified Southern Ontario winters. Gelled with an Arctic air mass and scattered with snowflakes, its colour palette did not extend beyond grey in all its shades and hues: the slate of the barren earth, the slick charcoal of the asphalt, cinereous skeletal trees raising their branches to the pale silver sky. Ronald Reagan had recently become the fortieth president of the United States; I had no idea who the prime minister of Canada was. Poland had been in the throes of the Solidarity movement for the past seven months – coincidentally, since the day we had left Poland. We had languished for six months in immigrant limbo in Sankt Georgen, a hamlet nestled in the foothills of the Austrian Alps, while our refugee petitions and immigration papers were being processed by the Canadian Embassy in Vienna.

Those six months were the worst of my life. First, the uncertainty – we had no idea whether we would obtain Canadian Landed Immigrant status or if we would have to go to another country instead. Then the lack of money – after the dollars we had smuggled out of Poland ran out, my father attempted to work in a sawmill where he nearly lost the fingers of his left hand; and finally, the everyday rudeness of the owner of our gasthof that had led to two altercations with my father. We carried the shame of being stateless and living on the mercy of the Austrian government and the United Nations Refugee Agency. My former classmates in Poland were staging pro-Solidarity protests and participating in student strikes while I scrubbed toilets in an Alpine pensione.

It was in Austria that I had decided I would not be one of those Polish immigrants my mother had met when she visited Canada three years earlier – those who never learned to speak English properly, who attended the Polish mass at the St. Stanislaus church, shopped in the Polish grocery on Roncesvalles Avenue and banked their money at the St. Casimir credit union. I was not going to straddle the Atlantic with one foot in Poland and the other in Canada, waiting for the day I would return home wrapped in the glory of the immigrant success story. Instead, I would do everything I could to become Canadian, whatever "Canadian" was. For me, it meant speaking proper English, studying hard, reclaiming my best student status and getting into medical school. I was not going to waste time looking back. But my plans remained on hiatus as we waited for our immigration papers to be approved by a faceless embassy bureaucrat.

In Poland, at the end of grade eleven, high school students decided on the electives they would take in their final year of high school to prepare for university entrance exams. Before we left, I had wanted to study English language and literature. In Polish, I had loved giving novels and short stories a close reading, parsing their sentences and plots. I loved the history of Polish literature and language. In my English classes, I had loved learning a new vocabulary and grammar rules. I could see myself doing it for life. What I never dreamed of, though, was becoming a writer – one of those creative creatures who lived on a different plane of existence. That I could not aspire to.

➥

My Polish classmates were mapping out their futures while I polished parquet floors and scratched for groschen under the rugs in a hotel bar, a job that I had cajoled from the fat, gum-chewing gasthof owner. For months, I did not know where, or even if, I would attend school come September. To save myself from going crazy with boredom, I studied the Polish grade eleven biology textbook my best friend had sent me and read Somerset

Maugham's *The Painted Veil*, which an Austrian high school teacher had lent to me to improve my English. As I read, I underlined the words I didn't know with a straight line, and the ones whose meaning I managed to glean from context – a technique I had learned back in Poland – with a wavy one. Then, I wrote all of these words in a notebook and translated them using Stanisławski's two-volume English–Polish dictionary that we had managed to bring with us. Painstakingly, I copied down the phonetics and definitions of each word, then memorized them. Soon I became well-versed in the vocabulary of the privileged, early twentieth-century English that inhabited the Far East outposts of the British Empire: "tanned" and "ayah" were the first two words I remember looking up, followed by "tiffin."

I'd finished reading Maugham by the time we received our Canadian Landed Immigrant status documents from the Canadian Embassy in mid-February. A week later, our plane tickets arrived in a thick, cardboard envelope. Caritas, a Catholic charity, lent my father money for them but only enough to take us as far as Toronto – even though he'd said we wanted to go to Vancouver. "If you want to go to Vancouverzu you go to Vancouverzu. In Canada, you can do whatever you want if you have the money," said Mr. Borowik, an official at the Canadian Embassy, during our interview. He spoke haughtily, his Polish rudimentary, his intelligence limited, betrayed by the declension of the city name – anybody with brains knew that in Polish you didn't alter the endings of foreign city names. We didn't have the money, and that's how we ended up in Toronto on that frigid March afternoon.

In spite of my seven years of English classes, two of those in English immersion, and committing *The Painted Veil*'s vocabulary to heart – or maybe because of it – my English proved woefully inadequate for even the most mundane needs. At the time, Ontario Immigration housed new arrivals at the Waldorf Astoria Hotel on Charles Street in downtown Toronto. This hotel had nothing in common with its New York City namesake, as my father explained to me the evening that we arrived. The American one stood for opulence and luxury; the Toronto one was rundown, its single-pane windows painted with hoarfrost and its stained carpets an undecipherable colour redolent with the passage of others. In our room, a thin wall separated the sitting area from two double beds; there was no TV, but there was a kitchenette with rusted elements and a wheezing fridge sat on the other side of the sitting room. Stacked white towels towered in the bathroom, many more than I had ever seen at one time. These white, fluffy rectangles were piled three high, their intoxicating scent probably a combination of cheap detergent and bleach. A Pole who had arrived from Austria before us explained that in order to appear civilized, he threw them onto the floor and sprinkled water on the pile to show he had used them. "And that thicker, smaller towel," he said. "That's for the floor when you get out of the tub." I wondered how he had figured that out.

On our third day at the Waldorf, my mother sent me to buy lunch. "Go right from the hotel," she told me, "cross three streets, maybe four" – the concept of "city blocks" does not exist in Polish – "then turn right on Yonge Street, the busiest street. You'll see a big yellow 'M' sign."

I completely missed Yonge Street and the Golden Arches, and lumbered along Charles Street almost as far as University Avenue before I decided that a street lined with old stone buildings nested amidst tall linden trees was no place for fast-food restaurants. Little did I know that two years later I would be admitted to Victoria College and get to enter those stately portals. Shamefaced, I backtracked and located Yonge Street after what felt like hours. The McDonald's there exuded its signature deep-fried reek. I grew wistful, remembering the same aroma from Baltic seaside restaurants during childhood holidays. I took my place at the end of the single line snaking out from four cashiers – after years of lining up for food in Poland, I was a pro. Except that in Poland there would have been four separate lines, and those condemned to the slowest would look daggers at the lucky ones who moved along to secure their goods. By comparison, this was the height of civility. The single line feeding into four sales points impressed provincial, immigrant me.

When I reached the counter, my eyes settled on the silver flashing between the salesgirl's pink lips: metal wires caged her top and bottom teeth. The previous summer, in Poland, I had read *The Godfather*; now I flashed back to Connie Corleone's wired jaw, broken by her no-good husband Carlo. This poor girl's jaw must be broken, I thought. My heart beat wildly at such a crass display of Western degeneration. Eyes fixated on her mouth, I haltingly ordered three cheeseburgers. I was speaking English in Canada for the first time.

"Do you want French fries with that?" she asked, metal flashing.

"No. Not French fries," I said. "Just fries." I did not know what French fries were. The counter girl shrugged, stepped back to pick up three oily red pockets from under the heater and dropped them on the tray in front of me. I checked the contents – yes, those were the kind of fries I wanted.

"That's it?" the girl asked.

I had no idea what she meant. "I beg your pardon?"

"Is that it?"

I shook my head, my cheeks burning hot.

"Is this all you want?" the man standing behind me prompted.

Relief. "Yes," I said. "Yes, that is all I want." I paid for the order, barely able to tear my eyes from the girl's mouth, and squeezed through the crowd feeling stupid and deflated.

✒

On April 1, 1981, we moved into an apartment across from the Fairview Mall in North York. Its sixteenth-floor windows faced west over Don Mills Road and the balcony – almost a terrace – overlooked the Don Valley at Leslie Street, with Yonge Street buildings poking at the sky on the horizon. In Poland, only party officials would live in an apartment this size – three bedrooms and a living room, what a concept! The rental office wouldn't even consider renting us a two-bedroom apartment because the age difference between my sister and me – ten years – was too great. The apartment also had one and a half bathrooms and two walk-in closets, both not much smaller than my room in Poland. The rent was not cheap, but my father, flush with pride at his newly found contract job at Kilborn Engineering, with a yearly salary of thirty-three thousand dollars – which to us seemed like an absurd amount of money – signed the first and last months' rent cheques with confidence. My mother wrinkled her nose at the heavy foreign smells caught in the carpeted hallways – it would take me years to label them as cumin and cardamom – but even she approved of the apartment and liked the view. From my south-facing bedroom window, I could even glimpse a sliver of Lake Ontario, seventeen kilometres away.

It was in this room, furnished with an IKEA pinewood desk and bookshelves, that I spent my evenings and weekends studying. I registered at the nearest high school, Georges Vanier Secondary School, up on Don Mills Road. It offered high school courses in the semester system. Studying only four subjects for half a year and then switching to another four seemed strange to me. And the students chose their own courses? In Poland, everybody took the same classes in every grade, from the beginning of grade one to the end of high school; the only choice offered was between art and music, and that did not come until high school.

When I told the guidance counsellor that I wanted to study medicine – was that an eye roll or just my immigrant's paranoia? – she enrolled me in grade eleven biology, chemistry, math and English as a Second Language. I could read English without difficulty, obsessively looking up all the unknown words, and understood most of what was said, but expressing myself in English was a different story altogether. I would build an eloquent, complex sentence in my brain, grammatically correct and sophisticated, only to be betrayed by my tongue, lips and larynx as they refused to conform to the new vowels and clusters of consonants. It was as if I were gagged with an invisible muzzle.

At the time, I did not realize the full extent of the distress my muteness, my inability to communicate, was causing me. I felt deficient and stupid, handicapped in my search for high marks and acceptance. My personality seemed flat and boring in my broken English, and I missed my sense of humour. The need to communicate resides in the limbic system, the reptile brain of humans that is responsible for emotions. Neural and emotional changes ensue when the desire to communicate is blocked. This can happen, for example, in people with aphasia, a loss of speech that can occur after a stroke. But such alterations also take place in immigrants or, to a lesser extent, tourists who do not know the language of their destination.

My only means of expression were the letters that I wrote in Polish at least once a week to my friend Asia. There and then the floodgates opened. I would write four, five pages, sometimes more.

In English, I remained functionally mute for two more years, and many more had to pass before I was able to play with words and phrases again. Even now, when the correct word materializes in my mouth, I am amazed that I can express myself effortlessly in English. I never take the ability to communicate in any language for granted.

Back at Georges Vanier Secondary School, during my first test in chemistry, I choked back tears. I knew the concepts, I knew all the answers, but I could not put them into English. It would not do. Good marks were the only connection between my old life and this new one I was embarking on. I waved the teacher over.

"I know the answers," I whispered, my voice shot through with panic, "but I do not know how to write them. I do not know the right words."

She pulled up a chair beside me and wrote my answers down, transcribing my half-verbal utterances into proper English. I got an A-.

On the other hand, Mr. Curlew's biology tests were much easier – a list of fifty questions that required only one-word answers. Once I figured out how his tests worked, I spent hours pacing my room, memorizing the biological terms. "Platy-hel-min-thes," I muttered, pronouncing every word as if they were written in Polish, to memorize their spelling. "Echi-na-cea." I received a perfect mark on the first biology test in his class.

Based on the fact that I had finished grade ten in Poland, an educational assessor at Ontario Welcome House, who never laid eyes on me, granted me twenty-four credits toward my high school progress and recommended that I start in grade eleven in September. At the time, a minimum of thirty-six credits was needed to graduate with an Ontario high school diploma and there was still a grade thirteen. At that rate, I would finish high school two years after my Polish classmates. Unthinkable – I, the brilliant grade-skipper, the best in my class all through primary school, would lose two years? I was heartbroken for days.

After the second biology test, which I aced yet again, Mr. Curlew pulled me aside and asked me about my plans for the following year. My anguish spilled out.

"They don't realize how much further ahead Polish schools are," I said. "If I had stayed in Poland, I would graduate high school next spring. All my friends are going to university next October."

A few days later, my guidance counsellor called me to her office. She said that I had impressed my teachers with my hard work and knowledge, and they had decided to grant me full credits for the half-semester in each of the four courses I was taking. If I took two full courses in summer school, she suggested, I would have enough credits to start grade thirteen in September.

"You could take six grade thirteen courses next year and finish high school. But you'd have to work very, very hard. And you'd have no summer holidays," she said.

Who cared about holidays? I'd had a six-month "holiday" in Austria following my regular summer holiday in Poland. Of course I was going to do what she suggested.

Later that year, I came across an impassioned letter Mr. Curlew had written. He described how I excelled in his class and requested that I be granted full credits for his biology course. He must have canvassed my other teachers – the letter bore their four signatures. I can still see his kind face, a halo of greying hair around his balding dome. But I never saw him again, and I never thanked him.

✒

That summer, I took grade eleven physics and English; no more ESL courses. I got credits for both courses, although only a B- in English, and was set to begin grade thirteen at the same time as my Polish classmates started their last year of high school. I would graduate with them – everything was right with the world again.

In September, upon the advice of our family doctor, Dr. Irene Abramowicz, I enrolled at York Mills Collegiate Institute. I signed up for six grade thirteen courses – functions, calculus, algebra, biology, chemistry and physics – as well as grade twelve English and grade nine Latin; I knew that I needed to know Latin for medicine. No spares.

Two weeks after school started, I was called to the nurse's office. She injected something under the skin on the inside of my left forearm. Overnight the puncture swelled to the size of a walnut; it throbbed and itched. The next day, I was called back to the nurse's office, where she stepped away from me, her eyes goggling, as I rolled up my sleeve.

"Go see your family doctor," she said. "You must get a chest X-ray. It looks like you have tuberculosis." She never told me what the needle prick had been for.

"Małgosia has tuberculosis. It's all your fault," my mother announced to my father that evening even before he took his coat off. "She must have gotten it in Austria. All those Asians at that Traiskirchen." We had spent two nights at the former Austrian army barracks–turned–refugee camp when we defected the previous summer. My mother had never wanted to leave Poland, and she and my father argued about it for years before she relented. My father had travelled to Vancouver on three business trips in 1976 and 1977 as a consultant on the construction of a coal-burning power plant in British Columbia. He'd fallen in love with Vancouver's snow-capped mountains, reflected in the indigo bay, and with the redwoods in Stanley Park. He had seen how Canadian professional engineers lived and realized he would never achieve that standard of living in Poland – although a member of the Communist Party, he was not cynical enough to advance by nepotism and sycophancy. Or maybe he simply did not want to.

He had joined the party as a first-year university student, a son of a poor farmer, idealistic and hopeful for the future, but fifteen years later he saw through the lies: a trough hogged by the fattest and the least scrupulous preventing those outside the cabal from getting even a sniff. And even though by Polish standards we lived a privileged life – a walnut-brown Polish Fiat 125p that few others could afford, a three-room apartment with a wall-mounted telephone, skiing in the Tatra Mountains, summer on the Baltic coast and even summer holidays abroad on the Black Sea – he'd had enough. But he had not imagined what we would have to go through before we reached Canada.

That evening in Toronto, my father's face paled, turning a chalky white at my mother's words, but I did not worry. How romantic, I thought. Consumption! Just like all those nineteenth-century poets and composers, like Ruby Gillis in *Anne of Green Gables*. Even though I knew tuberculosis was treatable with antibiotics, I imagined I would get interestingly thin and pale, like Dumas's *La Dame aux Camélias*.

But when I went to see her, Dr. Abramowicz told me I didn't have TB.

"You were vaccinated in Poland and the BCG vaccine causes the skin reaction," she said. "The nurse should have known. But you do need an X-ray so I can prove that you're not infected."

At that time, York Mills CI, nestled among the mature trees on a block between Leslie Street and Bayview Avenue, catered to the very privileged, mainly Jewish, neighbourhood kids, and to the academically gifted who arrived every morning from across the city. When I started there, I had no clue what the Lacoste crocodile that graced almost every polo shirt in the hallways signified. LeSportsac was the bag of choice. In an attempt to belong, I went to Holt Renfrew at Fairview Mall to buy at least a LeSportsac pencil case. It cost eighty-nine dollars for two flimsy pieces of plasticky fabric stitched together and topped with a zipper. Sanity and an empty wallet prevailed, and I went home to study instead – the only status I cared about was that of a class keener.

My home form and grade twelve English teacher was Miss Anglin. She was five feet at most, stout, wore manly jackets and squinted behind thick glasses.

"Is this school really so good?" I asked the morning I met her, in a perfect imitation of my father's arrogant tone.

"It has very high academic standards," she answered icily.

I probably deserved that answer.

She had no patience with me. The grammar she taught had nothing in common with the grammar I had studied in Poland. What was a predicate? Adverbial clause? Phrase? My classmates had learned English sentence structure in lower grades. I floundered, alone, in an ocean of ignorance. My limited English also prevented me from communicating any understanding of literary texts; only once did I manage to say why Shakespeare had described the clothes Duncan and Macbeth wore in such detail.

"Yes, yes, it was to convey rank," Miss Anglin cut my ramblings short.

When we discussed *Heart of Darkness*, she took offence at Conrad's use of the word "moustaches." "Immigrants," she said. "They may become bilingual, but their English will never be idiomatic." I took it personally – not only because Conrad was Polish but also because I was the only non-English-speaking immigrant in the class.

In other courses, however, I soon found my footing. I studied like a maniac, every evening for six to seven hours, and all day and evening on weekends. I quit my summer bakery job in order to concentrate on my studies. I fought for every percentage point in every grade thirteen course I took. Never before had I felt or been more alone. I made no friends. Was it because of my poor English? Because I was fat? Between stuffing myself on chocolate bars in Austria and on Canadian cold cuts never available in Poland, I had gained twenty-two pounds and had the beginnings of a second chin. I believed that people avoided me was because I was a recent immigrant.

I wished with my whole heart to become a Canadian and to belong, but I wanted to keep some of my old identity. One way to do that was to keep my original name, so I always introduced myself as Małgorzata. With the desperation of a recent immigrant, I thought, If I could learn a whole language, they could at least learn to pronounce one word. Since Małgorzata has the same etymology as Margaret – the Greek word "margaritos," "pearl" – it would have been an easy switch. But I wanted my name. "Maw-goh-JAH-tah," I answered when asked my name, the "j" the sound that begins the French "jamais." "Oh, it's so pretty!" Canadians would say, which always made me cringe – even in Polish, the sounds were rough, the "j" a bristle on a polysyllabic caterpillar. And, no matter how many times I enunciated it, it never sounded right on non-Polish lips.

At school, I ate my lunches alone. I rode the bus by myself, laden with textbooks and notebooks. Nobody talked to me except in class. Nobody seemed to care about me. I comforted myself with my near-perfect marks and my dreams of university and medical school. Like Mr. Curlew the year before, my grade thirteen chemistry teacher asked me about my plans, but his response was the polar opposite to that generous man's. When I told this teacher that I wanted to become a doctor, he proclaimed that getting into medical school was near impossible and pontificated about how all new immigrants wanted to be doctors.

☛

In my enforced English muteness, I missed telling jokes the most – those one-line zingers that I'd been notorious for back in Poland. I tried once, but I mispronounced "lunatic" so badly that my grade twelve biology classmates stared at me, bemused. A year later, having heard the word "jerk" on *The Love Boat*, I tried to use it ironically, but the expressions on my interlocutors' faces made it clear that I had once more botched the delivery. Several years later, when I attempted a pun that went over like a lead balloon, a colleague snarked, "It's obvious that English is your second language." But by then I could snap back, "Actually, it's my third."

I laugh much louder at jokes in Polish. They hit right in the middle of my being, just above my belly button. In an excellent essay, in Polish, on the conundrums of translating humour, Stanisław Barańczak, a critically acclaimed translator of Shakespeare, Donne, Dickinson and Ogden Nash, discussed working on a translation of "The Owl and the Pussy-cat," by Edward Lear. As I read about his linguistic acrobatics, the original elicited a smirk – it was cutesy. Barańczak finished the essay with the product of his labours and I guffawed – loud, uninhibited belly laughter. The Polish translation hit me right between the eyes; its apt hilarity went straight to my limbic system. Barańczak translated "and there in the wood a Piggy-wig stood" into "a hog sideways 'cross a road." The word "wieprz" conjured a vivid image in my brain of a male pig in all its snouty, stubbly, pink hoggishness, something that "hog" had utterly and completely failed to do. And it stood "sideways"; not just across a road but "sideways 'cross a road." English did not stand a chance. And I won't even mention the subtle irony and sophisticated humour of the Polish Nobel Laureate in Literature Wisława Szymborska – English translations do not do her poetry justice.

And Heffalump. I laughed myself to tears the first time my father read

Irena Tuwim's excellent pre-war translation of *Winnie-the-Pooh*. He choked on his laughter as he tried to read through his own hoots. The mere memory of "słoń – słoniocy!!!" (Piglet's squeals of "Heff, heff, heffalump") still tickles fifty years later. When I bought the English original, I went straight to the chapter "In Which Piglet Meets a Heffalump." It disappointed – none of that visceral humour, none of the tears of laughter materialized. More recently, *Czarci pomiot* sounded so much more menacing and sinister than *Hag-Seed*, Margaret Atwood's genius notwithstanding.

I still look up words in the English–Polish dictionary – not the battered, four-volume Stanisławski that has travelled with me from Poland through Austria to Toronto and Hamilton, and still stands guard on my bookshelf, but the easier-to-use and much more complete and idiomatic online dictionaries. Without fail, the Polish words are more immediate, more visceral. Intuitive, they elicit an emotional response in a way that English cannot.

For years, English remained a type of a code: it carried a one-to-one correlation with objects and abstract concepts, like an old-fashioned cable might, but it had no shades of grey, no overlaps between words. Only when I witnessed my sons learning to speak it did I realize that English was as organic as Polish. One could have fun with it just as I used to in my native tongue – you could make up words, mix up grammatical forms to create new meanings for puns and jokes, create diminutives. Hearing my son say "pitch white" or "Germanese," or telling me "to stop colding" him when I'd touch his belly with my icy cold hands, taught me more about English than years of speaking it. After many years in the borderlands of English, I finally have fun with it, too. Now my delivery is so self-assured, people don't dare attempt to correct my neologisms.

I read novels in English as soon as I could. John Irving's *The World According to Garp* had just come out and Miss Anglin had mentioned it in class. It was brutal – I had never read about child rape, transgender people or weird sex. Regular sex I knew about – it was well-described in the translations of *The Godfather* and George Bidwell's *Philip and Olivia*, which I had read late at night by the light of the street lamp outside my window as a tween. I searched for the steamy scenes, of course. But Garp's was an alien world. Every new chapter brought a new assault on my sensibilities, on my innocence. One morning between classes, as I curled up with it on the floor by my locker, Miss Anglin appeared by my side and asked what I thought about it, the one and only time she spoke to me directly. I did not know how to answer. Her beady eyes behind Coke-bottle glasses seemed to be laughing at me, as if she expected shock or outrage from a provincial immigrant. I told her that I liked it. But I wish I'd had somebody to debrief with, to decompress after reading it.

In the spring term, Miss Anglin handed out a list of Canadian writers for the Canadian literature segment of grade twelve English. I chose *Fifth Business*. Robertson Davies's subtle and wry humour impressed me. I picked up my ears when Liesl, the acromegalic giantess, explained to Dunstan the concept of "the twice-born" – people who changed their first names later in life. Just as Davies's protagonist changed his name from Dunstable to Dunstan, I would soon change mine to Margaret. In the following years, I read all of Davies's books, both his classics and those he was still writing. For years I yearned to speak like he wrote – an utterly unachievable feat.

With Monika for a name, my six-year-old sister never had the experience of watching people's eyes goggle when they tried to read her name. She spoke no English at all when she went to Forest Manor Public School, which we could see from our bedroom windows. One day in the late spring, my mother spied her building sandcastles all alone in the school sandbox during lunch. As she watched, nobody approached my sister. My mother was distressed when she told us about it at dinner, her voice shaking, but my sister seemed unbothered. I didn't give much thought to Monika, so preoccupied I was with my school and studying. She quickly picked up English and became best friends with a girl who lived in the apartment next door; soon, they were inseparable. She seemed to be doing much better socially than I was.

☛

I would have finished grade thirteen with much better marks if it weren't for the funny spell I went through the spring after my seventeenth birthday.

Suddenly, in mid-March, shortly after second semester mid terms, I lost interest in school so completely and so suddenly it was as if a switch had flipped. I couldn't study, couldn't concentrate. At first, I tried to push through, but soon I realized that it was futile – I just couldn't do anything. I even started to cut classes, staying outside on the school soccer field if the day was nice. I was blank, uncaring, all my motivation, my drive, my determination gone. Emptied of all desire, I felt like a limp, wrung-out rag.

On the one hand, I wondered what was happening; on the other, I couldn't care less. I just existed. Languished. Barely survived. I don't remember feeling guilty or anguished about it, I didn't feel sad – I just didn't care. Later, I would learn the term for it – anhedonia, an inability to feel pleasure – but at the time I believed it was caused by an innate, deep-rooted worthlessness that had finally been unmasked. I couldn't fool anybody anymore – I was a failure.

One lunch in May, I sprawled prone on the spring grass of a little parkette south of York Mills Road, a few blocks from my school, and languidly wondered what was going on. My apathy had lasted several weeks by then and still I didn't care. Why couldn't I study? Why was I not invested in my future? The loss of the driving force in my life didn't even register as worry; the realization dissolved as swiftly as it had materialized and I simply rolled onto my back in the grass and stared up at the passing clouds. I lay there, my mind blank and unperturbed like the surface of milk in a pan, until it was time to return for my afternoon algebra class where I gaped, uncomprehendingly, at the algebra equations that covered the blackboard. Though I remembered my father teaching me set theory back in grade one, now I couldn't be bothered.

Nobody noticed my state. My father had recently lost his job, an incredibly well-paying job that he had bragged he'd gotten by "just walking in off the street" when we arrived, so my parents had more important things to consider than the moods of their daughter. When economic tides turn, as I heard my parents discuss over and over again at the dinner table, immigrants and contract workers are the first to lose their jobs. My father was both. I was supposed to be the one thing they didn't have to worry about – the top student in any class. Of course I would be fine. My path was laid out straight as the arrow flies: study hard and everything would fall into place. It's just that I couldn't for some reason. Nothing seemed to matter. I felt worthless. I thought my lethargy was caused by a lack of a moral compass; I believed I didn't deserve any better than to fail at school and at life.

✒

In May, I was accepted to University of Toronto's Victoria College, my third choice after Trinity and St. Michael's Colleges. No scholarship offers, though, so I applied for Ontario Student Assistance Plan (OSAP) and received an interest-free loan and a bursary, just enough for tuition and textbooks. I would never have been able to attend university if not for that financial assistance. The money wasn't enough to cover living in residence so I commuted downtown by bus and subway two hours every day.

At university, I finally decided to switch my name to Margaret. After two years of being the officious Małgorzata, of having to explain how to pronounce my name and always hearing it said wrong back, I had had enough. I was disappointed Canadians hadn't picked a nickname or a diminutive they liked and called me that. In Poland, a nickname is given to you by someone as a part of the unfolding of a relationship, not the other way around. Nine years later, my best friend Nicolette (not Nicole, Nicola or Nicky; she only allowed her father to call her Nicky) explained that in Canada, you introduce yourself by the name you want people to call you. I wish I had known that – I might have chosen a different name. I did consider Margot but thought it too pretentious, Margaux even more so since I was not French. Maggie sounded too frivolous. Mags would have been nice, but I did not know it at the time. I could also have gone with the über-cool M.J. I never considered introducing myself with any of the Polish diminutives, like many women do after they emigrate – it felt childish.

My official documents – Landed Immigrant status papers, Social Insurance Number, high school and university transcripts, medical school diploma – belong to Małgorzata Nowaczyk, the Polish character "ł" not available in the typesets and typewriters of the 1980s, but I have been Margaret for thirty-five years now. My beloved husband of thirty years has always called me that. A few years back, I started to sign my emails "Marg" – it was shorter, faster and I liked it. But my American collaborators pronounced it like Homer Simpson's wife, with a soft "g," so I stopped – I am not Marge! Now, good friends do sometimes call me by a different name. They pick a funny nickname that colours our interaction for the moment – Mags, Maggie, Ma-ah-gret – the way my Polish friends still do. When a Polish friend phones and says, "Hi, Margot," I instantly know what mood he's in and that I should expect something different from when he greets me as "Gosia."

Despite changing my name, I remained friendless through my first year of university. Nobody was there to explain to me how the university worked, how to study and write exams, how to optimize marks. Had I stayed in Poland, I don't think that I would have become so competitive and afraid. In Poland, students were accepted into medical school directly after finishing high school – there was none of the insane competitiveness of North American pre-med years. My best friend Asia was planning to sit the entrance exams for dentistry, and I am sure that we would have studied together in the final years of high school, preparing. Although a personal statement and curriculum vitae were required as part of the medical school application package, all pre-meds knew that acceptance rode almost exclusively on marks. Because I had done so well in grade thirteen – at least at the beginning – after essentially no school for a year, I'd thought university would be easy, too, especially after I received ten out of ten on my first chemistry quiz. I seemed to have forgotten how hard I had worked for my marks the previous winter, and about that funny spell I'd experienced at the end of high school.

Like every September since grade one, I was excited for the new school year. I loved the smell of new textbooks and blank, fresh notebooks ready to be filled. I did not know that Physics for Life Sciences was the hardest of the non-major physics courses to take. So, of course I took it – medicine was a life science, after all, and I wanted to do things right, no shortcuts. I struggled horrendously. I also chose a higher-level calculus course because it was the prerequisite for the second- and third-year courses in the Biochemistry

Specialist program, my fallback if I didn't get into medical school.

I confided in no one – I was convinced that everybody I met was competing for the same few seats in medical school. I overheard classmates compare marks way above mine and I burned with envy. When they discussed minute points on exam papers that broadcasted their mastery of the subject without having to yell that they got a ninety-eight, I willed the floor tiles to open up and swallow me. I scrunched up inside, and the carapace that had begun to develop as a child, when my mother constantly criticized me, calloused even further to protect me from my classmates.

When I received a mid-seventy on my first calculus exam, I was so distraught that I lost my way on the subway, boarding the westbound instead of the eastbound train at St. George Station. I huddled in the door well, flattened against the sliding doors by the bodies of oblivious commuters, and cried soundlessly, sweating in my winter coat, gasping the stale and overheated air. I would never get into med school; how could I have been so arrogant as to think that I might? I was a good-for-nothing failure and would never amount to anything.

I realized I was on the wrong train only when the subway rolled into Spadina Station, but I could not get past the tightly packed bodies. When I stumbled out at Bathurst, I slumped down on a red bench on the platform. I don't know how long I sat there as trains lumbered by and rush-hour crowds thronged in and out of subway cars. Finally, I climbed the stairs to cross the tracks and board the westbound train to Bloor/Yonge, and then north, back home.

By the end of my first undergraduate year, my father was driving a teal-and-orange Beck Taxi in Toronto's east end every night, including weekends. His second contract position as an engineer had ended abruptly when a private design firm folded a few months after hiring him and he decided that he would not beg for another job. There weren't any – it was 1983 and the recession was in full force. My father's pride demanded that he do things his way. When his unemployment insurance ran out the following year, after a lot of soul-searching, my parents signed up for welfare. A social worker came for a home visit and approved our family for benefits, but by that time – possibly as a result of the humiliation of merely allowing the visit – my father had decided that he would not accept charity and started to drive the cab for even longer shifts.

That first year at university, I tried to study, I really did. I crammed biology facts and physics and calculus equations into my unyielding brain, but without success. It was a constant game of catch-up, a catalogue of missed targets. In the end, my GPA that first year missed the magic 80 percent average by 0.2 of a percentage point.

☛

But sometime during the summer after first year the sky began to shine again. The linden trees on campus blossomed, their heady sweet scent reminding me of Polish summers as I sat under them and read, my English finally good enough for literature. I devoured *The Plague* and wished that I, too, could be the only physician in an epidemic-ridden city. *The Magic Mountain* only added to my romantic dreams of medicine. When September arrived, I was raring to go – keen to put in the hours, to cram like I had back in grade thirteen. I began studying at Robarts Library, that enormous grey monstrosity on St. George Street. A joke from Poland: Who is the happiest man in Warsaw? Answer: The night guard at the Palace of Culture and Science, because he doesn't have to see it every morning. The palace was a thirty-storey Stalinist blotch on pre-war Warsaw architecture, turreted and pillared, held up by social realist statues of peasants and factory workers. The same joke could be said about Robarts.

I rented a one-and-a-half-cubic foot book locker on the twelfth floor in the yellow section of the stacks, coincidentally the home of Czech, Russian and Polish fiction, and staked out a carrel and a west-facing windowsill in which to study. On weeknights, I would call it a day at 10:00 p.m. and begin my one-hour trek on public transit back to Sheppard and Don Mills. Every Saturday, I arrived when the library opened at nine and left when it closed at five. On Sundays, my father drove me to Robarts for its 1:00 p.m. opening so that I could study there until 10:00 p.m. Saturday evenings and Sunday mornings were the only times I didn't study. On the subway and on the bus, I read or reviewed facts jotted down on index cards. During the week, I filled any free time I had with studying. I had become one of those super-keeners.

Writing was how I studied: I wrote the material out, over and over again. Since there were no oral exams in my undergraduate courses, I had decided that writing out the answers would help with answering questions quickly and correctly during exams. I was going to flood the exam booklets with quantity and quality. Every day, I wrote from memory what I had studied the night before. I covered pages and pages with thermodynamics equations in physical chemistry; with amide, ester and ether syntheses in organic chemistry; with statistical formulae. On rough yellow paper pads, bought for $1.80 at the Bookroom, and with a cheap, medium-point, blue Paper Mate pen I scribbled and scrawled. I bought narrow rule pads that fit in more material per page to save money. Writing longhand from memory reassured me, gave me comfort – if not in the knowledge acquired than at least as a tangible reminder of the effort and hours I had put in. My mistakes glared at me, blue on yellow, indelible – proof of my ignorance and stupidity. Sheets and sheets were filled with minuscule handwriting, a separate pad for each subject. The Polish idiom for such handwriting is "maczek" – "tiny poppy seed" – because the letters resemble strings of tiny black seeds lined up on the page. In addition to coagulating the knowledge in my brain and in the muscles of my right hand, and rewiring the connections between them, the physical act of looping the letters, stringing them into words, punctuating them with commas and periods and semicolons had a soothing effect.

Graphomania, also known as hypergraphia, is the frenetic activity of writing, often without meaning – the filling up of reams and reams of paper, notebook after notebook, sheets, sheaves, rolls. My graphomania began innocently enough as I wrote letters from Austria to my best friend, Asia. I tried to fit as much information as possible onto the pages of flowery paper that came with the stationery box I had bought. It was a utilitarian impulse – I didn't have enough money to buy another set, so I crammed the sheets with thousands upon thousands of characters two to three millimetres high. I saw nothing wrong or unusual in this – I was simply saving paper.

And now, this ability to write for hours at a time and on dozens of pages came in handy in helping me study. Or at least I thought so.

That year, I also started to volunteer at Humber Memorial Hospital where Dr. Abramowicz's husband was head of the pathology department. I watched him while he dissected organs and reported on surgical biopsies, and I learned the workings of a diagnostic chemistry laboratory. One Friday afternoon in late September, he sent me to the fluoroscopy suite to watch a percutaneous needle biopsy of a lung. Standing outside a large one-way window, I saw a woman's round pink back exposed under a large X-ray tube suspended on a metal arm from the ceiling. Overhead, a TV screen projected a black-and-white image of her ribs and blood vessels, and her beating heart. (Yes, just like in that scene in *The Magic Mountain* where Hans Castorp witnesses the beating of his cousin's heart!) A silver needle advanced from the top toward a round shadow behind the ribs, paused briefly with the tip in its middle, and then retracted out of sight. I didn't see much more than that because suddenly my vision narrowed to a tiny tube, shadows pressing from all sides. I staggered into the hallway and slumped against the wall. Sliding along the tiles, I made my way toward a window where two nurses sat eating a late lunch. I just managed to reach the garbage pail beside them when I lurched and my lunch spilled out. I had no idea that a "coin lesion" was a metastasis from the liver or colon that signified an advanced cancer and probably wouldn't have cared if I did. All I could think about was that losing my lunch proved I was not meant to be a doctor.

"That means that you are going to be a *good* doctor," one of the nurses said as she handed me a paper towel to mop my forehead.

My first university exam that year took place just after Thanksgiving. Physical chemistry was the toughest course I took that year and a prerequisite for my biochemistry specialist degree. I felt well prepared, and when the exam ended, I thought I had done well. The following Monday, marks were posted on the wall of the first floor of the chemistry building, outside the undergraduate laboratories. I found my nine-digit student number, a number that I will remember even in my most demented state at the end of my life – and read "66" next to it. My future flashed before my eyes: I was a failure. No matter how hard I studied I would never get into medical school.

I slammed my right fist into the taupe wall tiles under the notice. In spite of my fury, I managed to restrain myself enough to run out before I tore the sheets off the wall. But as the cool night air soothed my throbbing hot cheeks, I wondered about other students' marks. "Maybe it's so bad that the prof will have to bell it up," I thought. I couldn't have done *that* badly. I skulked back into the building to test my theory. I noticed no eighties or nineties as I scanned up and down, and a glimmer of hope flickered in my heart. Then I saw it – the mark listed was out of seventy-five. Sixty-six meant that I had gotten 88 percent. In physical chemistry, the hardest course I was taking that year.

I knew then and there that I would make it – I had figured out how to study, how to take exams and how to get the marks that would guarantee my admission to medical school. The remainder of that year was a whirl of studying, writing assignments, studying, tests, studying, quizzes, exams, studying. That winter, I met George, a Jewish-Hungarian immigrant with whom I shared memories of May Day parades, Lenin monuments and the glorious Soviet Union – the fixtures in our childhood universes. We regaled ourselves with tales of our passive resistance to studying Russian in both public and high schools, and soon realized that we loved the same Polish and Russian science-fiction writers from whom we quoted at random. He also wanted to become a doctor; in fact, he had been accepted into medical school in Budapest the summer his family decided to emigrate. His family went through the same immigrant limbo as mine before they arrived in Canada; theirs took place in Rome. At Robarts, we studied at the same table, ensured we did the assignments on time, quizzed each other on minutiae of organic chemistry and statistics, and edited each other's essays. But neither of us really knew what to expect beyond medical school admission.

Every evening, after dinner at the Formica-topped cafeteria tables on the first floor of the library, one of us would scoop up a discarded copy of the day's *Globe and Mail* and open it to the comics page: the highlight of our day was guffawing over the *Far Side* cartoon. If it was a really good one, I tore it out and put it between the pages of my organic chemistry textbook – they are still there.

I finally had somebody who cared about me.

But this was also the year I began to grade myself. Whenever I got a question wrong, I wrote "PAŁA" in the margin of the textbooks, partly to mark the spot that I needed to return to in my revisions, but mainly to admonish myself for what I considered a failure. "Pała" is a crude Polish word for police baton but in Polish students' vernacular it also stood for the dreaded "deuce" – a failing grade. There were only four grades: 5, very good; 4, good; 3, satisfactory and 2, a fail. There was no 1. It had been drilled into me from grade one onward: I needed to get 5s. All the time. Anything below a 5 constituted a failure. Brains were everything. Don't be shy about yours, my parents always told me. Get 5s and everything will be fine.

I had received my first pała in the dead of winter in grade one. Our teacher had announced the homework standing at the back of the class, rearranging our artwork pinned to the wall mats – I still remember that – and I had not registered her instructions. I wasn't the only one to miss the assignment – six others also got big, fat 2s. When I came home that day and told my mother about it, she went ballistic: How could I? I would never amount to anything! I was worthless, useless, good for nothing.

"Don't you ever bring home another deuce, do you hear me?" still rings in my ears.

I ended my second year of university with As in botany, organic chemistry, statistics and French, and an A+ in organic chemistry, my favourite course that year. But my 90 percent average was not enough to compensate for the poor showing in my first year: I did not get into any of the medical schools I had applied to. My marks, however, garnered me an NSERC summer research scholarship in a botany laboratory where I studied cold resistance in green algae and where, come July, I watched with envy as my classmate Martin stacked his first-year medical school textbooks after receiving his acceptance letter to University of Toronto Faculty of Medicine. George, whose second-year marks were lower than mine, received an offer of admission at the University of Ottawa and was wait-listed at the University of Toronto. I did not even place on a waiting list: all of my letters were outright rejections.

It took another year of cramming and churning out A+ marks to get into medical school, but I was happy that year; I knew my hard work was paying off. And whenever I felt dejected, George would shore me up on the phone and remind me how smart I was. In third year, courses were harder, exams more difficult to ace, and I bemoaned each percentage point lost. I switched out of a second-year French course, because it was obvious that I would not get the marks I needed; instead, I enrolled in the introductory Polish literature course taught by Professor Louis Iribarne, who translated into English some of the Polish science-fiction novels and short stories George and I revered. It was meant to be a bird course, the first I had ever allowed myself to take, but it ended up being much more difficult than I expected. I needed to write essays in English – on Polish literature, no less! – and my essay-writing skills were non-existent.

That year I also met Robert, George's best friend. We took a third-year human physiology course together and I helped him with second-year statistics, which George and I had taken the year before. He, too, was Jewish, but Canadian-born, and wanted to go to medical school but planned on getting his bachelor's and maybe master's degrees first. He was insouciant, carefree, and his wicked intelligence was coupled with the driest sense of humour I had ever encountered. He also spoke French fluently, something I had always wanted to be able to do, and freely corrected my English pronunciation and grammar. But even he was stunned when I asked him whether the English word "lousy" came from "louse" – it had never occurred to him. And I had to drag him to the *Oxford English Dictionary* that stood on a lectern in the reading room at Robarts before he accepted my claim that "a lot" was two words, not one.

As the year passed, Robert became more and more important, and before the end of third year I broke up with George and began dating Robert. He was nothing like George, nowhere near as kind or caring or solicitous. But I revelled in his humour and his attention, however fleeting and half-hearted it was – or maybe precisely because it was fleeting and half-hearted. I had a hard time pinning him down to his promises and he often had other things to do than to meet with me, but when we were together, I laughed a lot.

In spite of these romantic entanglements, my marks stayed steady. I finished third year with an A average again and received an early admission offer from Ottawa – I never knew such a thing existed – in mid-May. By that time, I was in the midst of an NSERC summer research project studying the taxonomy of salivary proteins in the laboratory of Dr. Anders Bennick. Accepting Ottawa's offer required payment of a non-refundable $150 fee, a huge sum of money for my family. Worried about the expense, I asked Dr. Rob Murray, a professor in the lab next door who taught biochemistry at the Toronto medical school, whether there was any way that I could find out earlier if the University of Toronto was considering giving me an offer. Kind Scotsman that he was, he walked with me to the Student Affairs Office at the Faculty of Medicine to inquire.

"If I accept the Ottawa offer, I have to pay a hundred and fifty dollars," I told the assistant who met us.

"There are people who would pay a hundred and fifty *thousand* to get into U of T medical school," she trilled.

I opened my mouth to say something that I would probably regret, but Rob grabbed my elbow and steered me away. He looked as shocked as I felt.

"You'll just have to wait, lass," he said as we walked down the corridor. "Sorry about the money."

I paid the fee, knowing that if I were accepted into Toronto, I would eat the cost.

✒

And then the day came: the University of Toronto's Faculty of Medicine was "delighted to offer me a position" in the incoming medical school class. Even though my entire life had just changed, I still had to finish my experiments that day. One of my duties was collecting saliva samples from donors among the graduate students. Dr. Bennick had rigged tiny cups the size of today's earphones via translucent tubes to a tiny suction machine. The whole apparatus was cobbled to a stainless steel cart that I wheeled from lab to lab asking for volunteers. A graduate student in an adjoining lab dubbed it the "spitmobile."

That wonderful, marvellous evening, after rinsing and sterilizing the spitmobile and closing the lab for the day, I sauntered toward University Avenue and hiked up the old Lake Iroquois incline of Avenue Road to the St. Clair subway station. Birds rioted in the soaring elms, the air scented with linden blossoms (my favourite smell), the day's humidity finally burned off – a Toronto summer evening in its full glory. My quest was over. The rest – finishing medical school – would be easy.

No fickle economic downturns would affect me: I would never be unsure where next month's rent would come from. Anyway, who needed rent – I would buy a house, my own house with stairs and a laundry room. I would have a whole room devoted to the purpose of washing clothes and linens. In Poland's tiny apartment buildings, we had no such luxuries – a tiny front-loading washing machine stood tucked into the corner of our minuscule bathroom; the contractor who tiled the walls had to chisel a four-inch niche so that the machine would fit. And a dryer, I would have a dryer. We had no dryers in Poland. A communal drying room in the basement with ropes strung from the ceiling served the whole building; my mother borrowed the key twice a month to hang our towels and bed linens. I would run between the fresh-smelling sheets and wrap myself in them as my mother scolded. We hung clothes to dry in the window or on the balcony in warm weather; on the heating elements in winter.

After medical school, I would air-dry my bedsheets on a clothesline in my own garden.

Over the next few days, almost all of the medical schools in Ontario – with the notable exception of McMaster University – offered me admission into their Doctor of Medicine programs.

2.

After my medical school admission, salivary proteins and the spitmobile were not that interesting anymore. I couldn't wait for the school year to start. My relationship with Robert shifted; he didn't want to hear about medical school. He scoffed when I ranted about *The House of God*, which was *the* novel read by medical students around the country – a ruthless exposé of the hypocrisy of American academic medicine in the 1970s. It was a brutal novel about the inhumanities of internship in a teaching hospital within the Harvard Medical School system where attending physicians, only interested in academic advancement and financial rewards, were portrayed as bloody insensitive jerks without a shred of empathy for interns or patients. None of that interested Robert one bit. Instead, he regaled me with tales of his research projects. Still, it was an utter shock when he phoned me the Wednesday evening of my first week in medical school and announced that he didn't want to see me anymore.

That was orientation week. I had never experienced an "orientation" to anything. The second-years presented us with a spoof of a survival handbook ("not everything is as bad as *The House of God*") and explained the quirks of the Medical Sciences Building, a sprawling grey brutalist bunker with a weird architectural frieze at its top, which housed the medical school lecture halls and teaching labs ("that thing in the front is supposed to be a double helix," and "students have been known to vanish into the black hole of the histology lab"). We were assigned lockers and – based on an arcane, non-alphabetized schema – divided into groups in which we would spend the next three years of preclinical training. Classes started at nine in the morning and went until five with an hour's break for lunch. It was a full-time job, being a medical student.

The Tuesday of that first week, our group of ten descended to the dissection lab located in the bowels of the medical school building, guided by the ever-increasing reek of formalin. Our two instructors explained that the cadavers were people who had donated their bodies to science. They reminded us that we should accord them all the necessary respect and gratitude by studying hard and performing dissections diligently. Two of us from each group of ten would dissect each week – we had three mornings to complete our dissection, and on Thursdays we would present our findings to our classmates.

"You are responsible for the learning of your colleagues, so make sure you do it well," one of our instructors, a retired surgeon, admonished. I nodded eagerly – I would do the best I could. He then pointed to a pyramid of dark-brown wooden boxes stacked on the stainless steel bench by the wall. Each was about two feet long and eight inches high and wide. "These are your bone boxes," he said. "Find the one with your number on it. You may take it home, if you wish, but they must be returned by the end of the course in the same state as you got them. You will get your own skull next semester."

I found my box and opened it. Inside, on sponge padding, lay yellowish bones with maroon streaks marking their ends and edges. I recognized a few: the stocky, round ones with a hole in the middle and stubby projections on their sides were vertebrae; the thin, tightly arched ones, the ribs. I knew that among the jumble of longer ones were the arm and leg bones, but I didn't know their names or even their positions in the body. The bones were lighter than I expected; they lay in my palm as if full of air – as indeed they were – the marrow washed away in preparation of the specimens. Their surface was porous, full of tiny holes and crevices, rough in places where, as I would learn, muscles had been attached. I named my bones Charles.

As I fingered their landmarks and imperfections, I couldn't shake my disbelief – these were real human bones. I felt proud yet awed by the tremendous responsibility bestowed upon me with this battered wooden box.

As we investigated our bone boxes, we studiously ignored the bulbous shapes that lay draped in dull white sheets on six stainless steel, hip-high tables along the periphery of the room. These were the cadavers we would be dissecting. Nobody mentioned them, even as we each snuck furtive glances around the room. In high school back in Poland, I had heard stories about medical students fainting upon seeing their first cadaver, or running out of the dissection room and never coming back. Was that going to happen to me?

"Well, are you ready?" our demonstrator asked.

We lifted the white sheet and the stink of formalin swelled around us. I saw a pale, thin body, yellowish as if made of wax, its belly sunken, arms tucked beside; its head was wrapped in green surgical towels. We would never see her face even as we dived deeper and deeper into the crevices and secrets of her body over the course of the semester. A yellowed sheet covered her from the waist down, tucked in around her legs and hips. Accompanying notes explained that our cadaver was a seventy-eight-year-old woman who had died of metastatic pancreatic cancer. I poked at her forearm with a gloved finger – the skin was rubbery, barely yielding. Unnatural.

At the end of the year, all of the cadavers and their brains, which we would study in the second semester in neuroanatomy, would be buried during a dedicated ceremony attended by both faculty and students.

That afternoon, I walked to the subway with Peter, a fellow first-year. As we chatted along the Philosopher's Walk behind the Royal Ontario Museum, it came out that I had arrived in Canada only four years earlier. Peter stopped and extended his hand to me.

"Congratulations," he said.

"For what?" I asked, genuinely puzzled. I thought he was making fun of me.

"That's a huge accomplishment," he said. I scoffed – I didn't get into med school on my first try, I didn't get any scholarships, I wasn't accomplished. I was convinced he was being sarcastic.

☛

Medical school orientation culminated on Friday night with a party at the College and Bay Pickle Barrel. After morning lectures, the second-years had planned a scavenger hunt for us – also a new experience for me – and the winners were to be announced that evening. I threw myself into the hunt.

Among other items, the list included a sexy dessert and a signed pair of boxer shorts from an upperclassman. We scored a surprise twenty extra points because I procured our boxers from Dimitri, the orientation leader. I had run to the downtown Eaton's, bought a hideous green and orange checkered pair, and prevailed upon Dimitri to sign them.

For the sexy dessert, the guys in my group had decided on a white chocolate boob topped with a chocolate nipple, but the winning team – unsurprisingly predominantly female – presented an erect and fully functioning penis. They had threaded a piece of intravenous tubing down the length of a banana and, at the right moment, squeezed a solution of cornstarch through it. When the goop hit the ceiling, our team conceded: theirs was a feat of engineering if not medicine.

Although I thoroughly enjoyed the partying and finally being part of a group, on the subway home, like all evenings during orientation week, I was already studying the structure of the heart; I couldn't wait anymore. From anatomy – the structure of the body, its organs and their organization – to histology – the study of the microscopic structure of the tissues that make up organs – I couldn't wait to finally hit the books.

☛

I had been fascinated with the human body since I found my mother's *Mała Encyklopedia Zdrowia* (in English I call it *Little Encyclopedia of Health*) tucked behind other books on the shelves of my parents' bookcase. A compact, grey cloth-bound volume filled with tiny words printed on the thinnest paper I had ever touched. My mother pried it from my unyielding hands, saying, "You're too young for this." The one time I managed to sneak a peek, I noticed, deep in the book's gutters, the ragged edges of the stiff, shiny pages that bore photo plates. They looked like they were cut out with manicure scissors.

"What was here?" I asked.

"Terrible pictures I couldn't look at," my mother said. "I had to cut them out."

"Pictures of what?"

"Hydrocephalus and kids with other diseases. Awful."

I tried to imagine what hydrocephalus – "waterhead" in Polish – would look like, but I couldn't quite picture it and was scared of what I imagined. The photos must have been horrific for my mother to butcher the book as she had, I thought. Monstrous heads squirting water from their ears and eyes and nostrils popped into my imagination for weeks afterwards, especially at night. Several years later, I found an unmaimed volume on a neighbour's shelf and, my heart thumping in my throat, searched for the photos that had disturbed my mother so. I found a much less frightening image of a girl with an expanded skull sparsely covered with hair, and eyes with irises partially covered by the lower eyelid as if sunsetting. Our imagination's ability to outdo itself when we think of the unknown and the unseen, furnishing our minds with the most monstrous and horrific visions, would be something I would experience again decades later when I began caring for women in the prenatal diagnosis clinic.

By grade two, I was reading *Little Encyclopedia of Health* regularly, riveted by its detailed descriptions of organs, diseases and infections. I loved the line diagrams: clawed toes and crooked arms were rendered in pencil-thin detail; a series of cartoons depicted alcohol intoxication, the last frame showing a coffin; the eyeball and the inner ear drawn in cross-section – the snail-like cochlea and the layers of the retina reminded me of Arras tapestries I had seen in the Royal Castle in Kraków. Sometimes, I ran my fingertip along the cut edges of the photo plates, not afraid anymore.

In grade eight, on a sunny and bright September morning, Mrs. Antończyk, our human biology teacher, loped into our fourth period class and asked for the textbook. When a boy handed her his copy, Mrs. Antończyk stood it on its spine on her desk and let it go. The book's covers splayed apart and its pages fluttered open to about two-thirds through. She chuckled.

"Whenever I pick human biology textbooks at the start of the year, they always fall open to the chapter on human reproduction," she said.

The class tittered.

"It's only natural," she said. "I'd rather you learn it here than on the street. But first we need to learn about cells."

And so began my favourite subject. Out came *Little Encyclopedia of Health* – by then tattered and missing its covers – from which I supplemented the meagre information found in the textbook. I read and reread the parts on the normal functions of body systems – circulatory, respiratory, digestive. They stuck in my brain. The diagrams of the skeleton, reminiscent of the medieval depictions of death and hell from my parents' art albums, were creepy at first, but soon I got over that discomfort. How the body worked and how everything in it was put together intrigued me; diseases, not so much. The encyclopedia didn't discuss treatments or therapies; it was a book about health.

On a class trip that November, in a bookstore tucked into the side of Kraków's cobblestoned medieval market square, I spotted a colour atlas of human anatomy much more detailed than either our school textbook or my mother's encyclopedia. I bought it on the spot, ferreting small coins from my pockets and wallet. The diagrams of heart valves and the lobes of the brain were much more captivating than St. Mary's Basilica or the Wawel Royal Castle. I pored over the slim volume for two hours as the school bus rattled back to Gliwice, my hometown.

On the first test Mrs. Antończyk gave us, I described the structure of the eye in such detail that when the bell rang, I had only answered the first of four questions. I was sure the bell had malfunctioned. Or that it was a fire alarm.

"The period's over," Mrs. Antończyk said, standing over me, her hand out to collect my answers.

"But I didn't finish," I wailed.

She took the paper from my hands. "That's just too bad," she said.

When she handed out the marked papers later that week, the first page bore a red, circled "5," with "Don't dawdle" scrawled across the top. I looked up to see her smiling at me.

That spring, the Polish Ministry of Education had instituted the "report card with the stripe." It was actually a thin red-and-white Polish national flag that ran from top to bottom on the ivory-coloured certificate, but we always referred to it as "the stripe." It distinguished the student with the highest marks at graduation. A nickel-plated pin accompanied it – half

Polish Eagle, half open book. When the principal introduced the award during our graduation ceremony, my heart sank – I knew, I just knew that my classmate Ewa would get it. Her marks were as good as mine and she was the best-behaved student, put up as an example to me every time I screwed up. Ewa received the Exemplary Student badge every term, meanwhile my conduct was never considered exemplary. If I had a good semester, I would get Outstanding, the second-best designation, but most of the time my conduct was just Good. I was trouble, I misbehaved, I interrupted the teachers with questions. To boot, I was an uncoordinated klutz and I never managed a 5 in phys. ed.

My mother was going to be so mad when she learned that I didn't get it.

"Małgosia Nowaczyk," the principal announced.

I got it! The first year it was ever introduced, I received the report card with the stripe – the only one in the whole school. My home form teacher had given me Exemplary in conduct after all, and the gym teacher had taken pity on me.

It was the last time I would be the best at anything.

☛

Seven years later, long after my struggles with high school English and first-year undergrad courses, I wanted to win the academic gold medal for the highest overall standing during medical school; to be the best again. I knew I had the brains to get perfect marks, I had finally figured out how to study for university-level courses and – most importantly – I was willing to put in the hours and the effort. I had the stamina and the tenacity. I was finally learning about what I had always wanted to study: the human body.

I had read about medical school's gold medal in Mordecai Richler's *The Apprenticeship of Duddy Kravitz* a year earlier. It was the traditional award bestowed on the student graduating with the highest average over the entire course of study. Duddy's brother Lennie – a brilliant student – was in the running for it before he allowed a well-heeled WASP classmate to plagiarize his work. Lennie was expelled and the classmate got off scot-free. If I ever get into med school, I promised myself at the time, I would go for the gold medal.

I had completely forgotten about that "funny spell" I had experienced, and I had not yet met the real geniuses of my class. One, also named Lennie, skipped lectures and then locked himself in the anatomy museum for two nights before the mid term only to emerge with a perfect mark; I managed an eighty-eight after studying for weeks. Or Ken who had the wickedest sense of humour and could recite entire biochemistry lectures from memory; he would end up the gold medallist in our class. I do not have an eidetic memory; I had to study and study and review and review to retain information, but when I did learn something, it stayed with me forever. Thirty-five years later, I still remember the osteoclast, a bone cell that resembles a tennis racket, and how vinca alkaloids extracted from the periwinkle plant interfere with cell division in cancer cells by blocking the production of intracellular microtubules required for cell division. I worked hard and studied longer.

I practically memorized almost one thousand pages of *Ham's Histology*, by Ham and Cormack, and tried to do the same – much less successfully – with Moore's *Clinically Oriented Anatomy*, but perfect marks eluded me in medical school. After over a hundred hours of studying and reviewing, I would get an A and be thoroughly disappointed. I scoffed at a classmate who said that all we needed now was "six-oh and go," because in medical school the passing grade was 60 percent. I still wanted to if not be the best then at least *do* my best.

I loved my courses. Histology – the study of tissues unaffected by disease – was held in the microscopy laboratory where every one of us was assigned a locker with a microscope and another wooden box, this one much smaller than the bone box and containing a hundred representative slides of healthy human tissues. Every single one was breathtakingly beautiful in its own abstract way. Adipocytes stacked like lilac balloons. Pale pink bones – those had to be decalcified before sections could be cut. The kidney's purple glomeruli, each resembling a tiny garlic bulb. I loved it all and soaked up the knowledge like a parched sponge. Every evening after classes, I sat in the histology lab reviewing the day's material and picking up glass slides at random from the box to test myself.

The medical school texts held me in thrall like the zoological and botany atlases of my childhood. Collections of exotic specimens to satisfy my curiosity: healthy and diseased tissues, human bones, muscles of the forearm and the hand, the plates of the skull, the ever-branching nerves and arteries. And even if embryology made me believe in a higher power – that something so intricate, so complex, so perfect and beautiful as the human body could arise from a single cell without any glitches as often as it did, was proof of the divine to me – in my mind, diseases were separate from people and their lives. Patients' social situations, the emotional underpinnings of illness, secondary psychological complications – the "psychosocials," as we dismissively called them at the time – held no interest. Who cared if a patient was married or how large their family was? The disease was always the same, the biological processes that held their body together didn't change if they were a boat person from Vietnam or a multi-millionaire with a glimmering Rolex and a Rolls Royce. Lawyers and miners and sex workers all ailed the same way, I thought at the time, even if they tended to suffer from different diseases. In the mid-1980s, the scientific model of disease reigned supreme. The body was viewed as a closed biological system that obeyed physical laws and as such could be manipulated with medications and surgery to return it to its original equilibrium. And while we were told that health was not simply the absence of disease, our teachers didn't dwell on other determinants of health.

To learn how the human body functioned, how it malfunctioned and about the biology of diseases – that was all I cared about. Curing disease came second. Anything else was fluff.

I continued my undergrad study habits, spending hours memorizing, writing and rewriting my histology and anatomy notes. Because I had majored in biochemistry, I was granted an exemption from the first half of the biochemistry course in medical school. That meant that the exam I would take at the end of the course would be worth 90 percent of my final mark. I couldn't mess it up. I had received full marks on the two laboratory assignments, so I could potentially get a perfect score in the course. And I had become hooked on medical biochemistry from the first lecture I had attended on a drizzly, darkening November afternoon after mid-terms.

In the cavernous lecture hall that fit our class of 252, Rob Murray lectured on galactosemia, a disease caused by the deficiency of an enzyme that digested galactose, the sugar present in all dairy products and breast milk. Galactosemia causes liver failure, cataracts and intellectual disability. A single enzyme deficiency caused dysfunction in three completely unrelated organ systems: the liver, brain and the lens of the eye. Amazing – what could be the common denominator?

So began my obsession with rare – "weird and wonderful" in medical student jargon – diseases. In a pocket-size, three-ring red binder, I recorded: Kallman syndrome, a lack of smell and underdeveloped genitalia; Alport syndrome, a combination of hearing loss and kidney failure; and many other eponymic conditions named after the men who discovered them. These seemingly random associations titillated my brain as I wondered about the underlying mechanisms that might tie together sex and smell, hearing and the filtering of blood. But our clinical teachers cautioned us against diagnosing the rarest of the rare diseases: "When you hear hoof-beats, think horses, not zebras," they said. In medicine, as in life, common things were common, so we should not jump immediately to the weird and wonderful. Except that *my* brain glommed onto the rare, eschewing the common cold, asthma or diabetes.

Robert's callous phone call during orientation had devastated me, but the breakup propelled me to study even harder, longer. Robarts Library welcomed me again for hours every evening and on weekends – I claimed the same carrel, the same book locker as in undergrad. By the end of the first term, I had prepared thoroughly for the anatomy and histology exams, and knew I had done well in both, but, as fate would have it, I ran out of steam just before the final biochemistry exam. In spite of having attended all the lectures and labs, and having taken copious, meticulous notes, by eight o'clock the night before the final I had done no reviewing. I was paralyzed with fear and incomprehension: How could I not be ready for my favourite subject? I had nobody to talk to – I never confided in my classmates, whom I viewed as competitors in a medal race.

So, I phoned the only person I could think of.

"What time is the exam?" Robert asked.

"Nine a.m."

"Pull an all-nighter."

I had never heard the term.

"It's when you stay up all night and study," he explained.

So I did.

For the first time in my life, I sat at my desk the entire night. I reviewed notes and kept myself awake by munching on wheat berries that had been meant for krupnik, my favourite soup. I chewed through almost a pound of them that night, crushing them between my front teeth. By the time I got to the last page of my notes, the sun had risen – a glorious pink and mauve January sky – and the insides of my lips and the tip of my tongue were raw. It was time to catch the Sheppard Avenue bus and then ride the subway downtown.

I wrote the exam as if floating underwater. There was no thought involved. My eyes read the problems; my hand filled out the circles on the multiple-choice computer card. Knowledge flowed through me – eyes-hand, eyes-hand, bypassing brain every time. I answered only one question wrong when the automatic neural connections began to fray. It was the second-last question on the exam: "What are the end products of glycogenolysis in the liver?"

My final biochemistry mark was ninety-five.

☛

In the new term, our subjects were neuroanatomy, pharmacology, physiology and interviewing skills, the latter being our first course held in the hospital clinics, with real patients. The introductory session of Interviewing Skills was held on the first Tuesday of the new term. Our anatomy group marched to Toronto Western Hospital through the slushy narrow streets of Kensington Market. Our class had been divided into groups sent to one of six teaching hospitals: Toronto General, Wellesley, Western, Women's College, St. Michael's and Sunnybrook. Once there, we were further divided into six-person groups. Jan (short for Janet), Douglas, Lesia, Susan, Eileen and I would continue together for the next two and a half years, attending clinics in the hospital first once then twice a week. In Interviewing Skills, we learned how to gather medical history from patients, the difference between open-ended and closed-ended questions, how to establish eye contact with a patient and how to put a patient at ease by matching their posture and speech patterns.

The word making the rounds among the medical students at that time was "empathy," taken directly from our course notes. I had never heard the term and yet I was required to not only understand what it meant but also to apply it in my interactions with patients. What was this beast called empathy? We were told that it was not the same as sympathy, that it required an appreciation of a person's predicament (what was that?) and putting ourselves into the patient's shoes (that phrase, at least, I did understand). I overhead classmates joking about it while I still struggled with the concept, so new and so alien. I knew sympathy – to feel with a person (from Greek, *syn* – with and *patheia* – feeling; yes, I did look it up in a dictionary in the hopes that its etymology would help me comprehend) – but this *em-* prefix threw the whole enterprise into an unreachable abstract. I realize now that the teachers had made it unnecessarily alien and academic instead of fostering our innate ability to feel for a fellow human.

In clinics, before we were set loose on patients who'd volunteered to participate in the course, we practised taking medical histories from each other. First, the instructor asked us to pick a colleague and describe his or her body language and what emotions it depicted. Everyone joked that they wanted to pick me – I was a cracked-open book. My clinic-mates most likely knew how much I wanted to excel and how much I resented their successes. But did they see how terrified I was as the term progressed and I fell further and further behind?

When we began interviewing real patients – as a group, under the supervision of the instructor – I was frightened to open my mouth, afraid of saying the wrong thing, of hurting the patient's feelings; of breaking them like a fragile ornament with a wrong word, a clumsy turn of phrase. I also worried about my ability to communicate in English – after all, only four years earlier I had been functionally mute.

My first interviewee was a man diagnosed with paranoia, hospitalized because of a psychotic breakdown. He was convinced that he was impotent because he was completely bald. Of course, we were not told any of that before I started to interview him – I was supposed to glean the information on my own. When he admitted halfway through our conversation that he wore a thick, black-haired wig, I was shocked. "Nobody knows about it," he said just before telling me that he had never had sex. Later, our instructor told us the patient had never admitted he was a virgin. She said that this confession was a "breakthrough in his care." I was flushed and shaking when the patient left the room, and became almost giddy when she said that. I realized then the power that simple words, used with care and respect, could provide.

I was probably overreacting at that moment, but after that encounter, my fear of talking to patients lessened, even if it didn't disappear completely. Each interview with a new patient was nerve-wracking – we never knew what we were going to get, what we were going to learn, what the patient might say. To add to the challenges of learning to work face to face with patients, we were being marked on how well we conducted our interviews, how we presented the cases and whether we got the diagnoses right. Even without the added pressure of marking, it was terrifying to walk into a room armed with a clipboard, a brand-new white coat and an earnest expression, and ask a complete stranger detailed questions about how their body functioned. Amazingly, all patients generously answered even the most intimate questions posed by this greenhorn medical student. Yes, we had to learn to obtain a sex history, too.

Back in the safety of the school, in the neuroanatomy lab, the brains that had been removed from the cadavers dissected in the fall awaited us in white plastic buckets, floating in formaldehyde – one brain for three students. My partners were Debbie and Rob. I don't remember dissecting the brain at all. I must have done some, at the beginning, because I do remember the rubbery feel of the fixed cerebral hemispheres with the spinal cord the width of my thumb peeking out from beneath the pleated folds of the cerebellum. Normally, the brain is soft like butter at room temperature and therefore completely unsuitable for dissection and study. It has to be fixed by soaking in formalin for several weeks before it can be handled without destroying its architecture.

It should have fascinated me. I should have been in there like a hog in a mud puddle, but instead, I read Tolkien. I had devoured *The Hobbit* during Christmas break and was onto *The Lord of the Rings* trilogy by the time the second term started. I read in the dissection lab as Rob and Debbie dissected next to me. Even when I wanted to catch up, the lectures in neuroanatomy did not follow the dissection schedule – they were system-based, and the dissection, by necessity, proceeded topologically from the outside in; it was almost as if they were two separate courses. As my partners dug deeper, they carved away the outer layers of the cortex and thus destroyed it, so there was no way to make up for the missed dissections. I floundered.

By March, I simply stopped going to neuroanatomy dissections altogether, and skipped physiology labs and most lectures.

I didn't realize what was going on until I saw a psychiatrist that February. Now, the funny spell I'd experienced had a name: clinical depression. The psychiatrist suggested that I try medication and prescribed amitriptyline, a tricyclic, one of the oldest antidepressants known to man and one of only two available at that time. I took it that evening and barely made it out of bed thirteen hours later. Staggering from the bus to the subway, I slept the entire ride from Sheppard Avenue to Queen's Park and then collapsed for the rest of the morning on a couch in the students' lounge. When I came to, it was afternoon and people were milling about, eating lunch and pretending not to notice me and my state.

I took the amitriptyline for about two weeks and then stopped. It was only making me sleepy, dopey, tired, and I was already having difficulty paying attention to lectures or studying in the evenings. But I continued to see the psychiatrist weekly – at least I had somebody to talk to about my worries and fears.

I don't remember any of my classmates asking me what was wrong.

Maybe they did. Maybe I lied and said that everything was okay. I'm sure I was too proud to admit there was anything wrong – vulnerability was not my strong suit, and I was afraid of being a failure. But I didn't realize how much I needed help.

A paranoid undercurrent seeped into my thinking: I was not appreciated because I had a funny surname and spoke with an accent. I did not get a medical school entrance scholarship or the summer scholarship I had applied for because I had an unpronounceable first and last name. I had no connections and no mentors; it was me, alone, against the world. My parents were no help – they knew nothing about medicine or studying it, nothing about how a Canadian university worked, nothing about my future plans and prospects. It never entered my mind that there could be others in the same position as myself – probably quite a few of my classmates were recent immigrants whose parents' dreams had not materialized. But finding out any of this would have required admitting vulnerability. Appearances had to be maintained; I pretended to be smart, successful, that I was doing great.

The term limped along. I tried to attend lectures, struggled to take notes. Physiology gave me the most trouble – I think if I had studied it the way I had studied everything in the past, I might have gotten all those intricacies and mechanisms down pat, but I did not even try. One frigid March morning, I simply did not show up for the physiology mid-term. I lied that I had been sick with the flu and the professors agreed to give me a makeup oral exam. A respirologist, an exercise physiologist and a cardiac electrophysiologist, all men, crowded in the respirologist's tiny office crammed with books and computer printouts stacked on his desk and shelves, asked me a few questions and gave me a seventy-five. I remember their puzzled looks when I showed up wearing a red beret that I did not take off for the duration. To this day I wonder why I kept it on.

I ached for friends. I longed for intimacy and the sharing of experiences – studying together, in-jokes – but had no idea how to make it happen. On an April afternoon in the physiology lab, one of the few that I attended, we conducted an experiment in which a subject was to breathe into a 150-litre balloon until it filled up and then we were supposed to measure the amount of the exhaled carbon dioxide. Susan volunteered to be the subject. After about forty minutes, she accidentally dropped the reed and, with a hiss, the balloon partially deflated. Red-faced from all the blowing and from embarrassment, Susan struggled to grab it but the experiment was ruined.

"Leave it to Susan to mess things up," I quipped. I meant it ironically – Susan was always careful and exact, she never made mistakes.

Cries of "How could you?," "That's not nice" and "Margaret!" erupted around me. I tried to explain that I did not mean it, but the damage was done. I was, officially, an insensitive jerk.

At about that same time, I started to knit obsessively. I brought my projects to classes and knitted and purled and cabled instead of taking notes in physiology and neuroanatomy lectures. I couldn't concentrate on studying or reading, so I looped yarn. I made replicas of the expensive Irish fisherman sweaters my classmates wore. At home, I sewed patterns by Ralph Lauren, Calvin Klein and Laura Ashley, and pretended they were the real stuff. I couldn't afford clothes from the brand-name stores, but I splurged on a Liberty fabric and Polo socks that might've suggested that my other clothes were the real deal – I wanted to appear as privileged as I imagined my classmates were. I did buy expensive shoes and leather boots, I couldn't fake those. I polished them daily and rinsed them in the hospital bathroom after every trek from campus to the hospital clinics through the salty winter slush. I had a blind spot for anybody who was not privileged – the peril of always comparing up – so I didn't allow myself to realize how many of my classmates came from a working-class background or, like me, were recent immigrants.

And so it went. I hated the feeling of not keeping up. I wasn't learning the material and I didn't know what was going on, but I wasn't going to let anybody know how terrified I was. My gold medal dreams were but a memory, as were any hopes for scholarships, but my ambition persisted. I wanted a residency at a top-notch institution like SickKids, Boston

Children's Hospital or Johns Hopkins. I wanted to work at a teaching hospital; to have an academic appointment, a university career. I wanted to be an expert respected by my colleagues; to publish papers and write textbooks. I wanted to keep going up and up.

How was I going to achieve all of this if I couldn't study? I was terrified that I would fail and distressed that my marks were slipping, but I kept pretending that everything was okay. Nobody was going to know how scared I was, how angry I was at myself for letting this happen yet again.

☛

But somebody did try to help the walking one-person disaster zone that was me.

"You ... you really don't need to study all this." The nondescript guy who had hunched over his microscope several seats behind me for most of the evening, now stood in front of me. He waved his hand over the brick that was *Ham's Histology*, ran his finger along my pencil underlinings, which covered the entire page. "Cormack's got all you need," he added, referring to the "histology lite" textbook by Ham's protege.

It was late November and I was still in the middle of my crazy studying routine, reviewing slides and notes in the histology lab after hours. I bristled at the interruption and looked up, straight into earnest brown eyes.

"Fuck off, I know what I am doing," I blurted. I did not add that I needed to be the best in the class. Best in everything.

The guy's cheeks reddened; he opened and closed his mouth. After a beat, he turned on his heel and slouched out of the lab without a second glance.

After ten that evening, as I swung around the corner to the locker room, arms full of textbooks and notebooks, I almost ploughed into him. We both stepped back. He looked ill at ease to see me, but I was glad I had run into him.

"Listen, I'm sorry about earlier," I said. "It's just – I am going through some really tough times. I was rude."

Many months – years? – later, he told me that he fell in love with my smile right there and then.

Jimm was a year ahead of me. Second-years used the same microscopes for their pathology work, but I had never noticed him in the lab before. After that disastrous beginning, he didn't approach me again. Once, I saw him studying with a girl from my year and I thought he should be hanging out with me instead – I was much prettier. When we passed in the hallways, we greeted each other but never talked – until one snowy, dark February evening when I asked him out for coffee after the Medical Students' Council meeting we had both just attended.

"Pathology mid-term tomorrow," he said by a way of explanation.

"After?"

"Sure."

The next morning, the moment I saw him in the cafeteria as I was getting my coffee, I regretted having asked him out – he'd showed up to school wearing droopy surgical green pants, a baggy maroon sweater with ragged cuffs and a hole over his left elbow, and a five o'clock shadow. Oh, well, it's only coffee, I thought. I did not want to make too much fuss. But that evening, when he returned to the histology lab where I was futilely trying to catch up on the neuroanatomy dissections I had missed, he appeared clean shaven and cologned, with a horrifically shiny, orange-red patterned tie knotted under his chin. And he wore a suit. He smiled sheepishly when he came over to my desk.

"I locked my keys in the car," he said, his cheeks pink. "It's parked out front, running. I have to dash home to get the spares."

He had made it into a date. With a really bad start.

An hour later, a moustachioed maître d' ushered us into the Mermaid on Dundas Street, directly across from the Art Gallery of Ontario. The smell of fresh fish broiled to perfection wrapped around me.

"My parents used to take me here for my birthdays," Jimm said.

Nice parents, I thought. "I love seafood," I said, taking in the dark wood-panelled room. Flickering tea lights danced on the snow-white table-cloths that covered every table. Cutlery and wineglasses clinked.

"They have a great selection of fresh fish," he said.

"I meant scallops and shrimp and lobster," I said, and immediately felt stupid and provincial. I had always thought "seafood" meant only crustaceans and molluscs, and did not include fish.

He ordered pan-roasted cod for me – I never knew fish could taste that good. We each had a glass of wine, a vintage suggested by our waiter. Over the crème caramel, I noticed what a manly square his chin cut against the Windsor knot of that awful tie. Hey, I thought, this guy's handsome.

The cheque arrived.

"Oh, no." I was to learn later that Jimm never swore, and he didn't then, either, but he did blanch. "I don't have enough money," he whispered, leaning across the table, the candlelight reflecting in his wide pupils.

"What?!"

"I have enough to cover the bill but not the tip. They've raised the prices since the last time I was here." He fiddled with his tie. "I cannot not leave a tip."

This guy has class, I thought as he rose and disappeared into the restaurant's kitchen.

After we left, Jimm and the maître d' exchanging apologies and reassurances, we had to scrounge around for money to get the car out of the parking lot at the Grange – we found enough in the glovebox and in our combined pockets. I directed him to a parking lot off Lakeshore Boulevard with a panoramic view of the downtown banks and the CN Tower. We watched the pale lemon-yellow disc of the sun rise over the battleship-grey winter waters of Lake Ontario.

I arrived home just after 8:00 a.m. to find out that my mother had phoned the police, who told her that they would not start searching for me until twenty-four hours had passed – she couldn't believe their callousness.

✒

After that, Jimm stuck to me like glue. On weekends, we studied in the empty classrooms of the Medical Sciences Building, but not together – we would commandeer adjoining rooms and visit each other every hour or so. In the microscope lab, students reviewed histology and pathology slides at all hours of the day and night; others claimed the smaller lecture halls and studied at the professor's desk, in front of blackboards covered in lists of drug side effects or nerve tracks in the brain stem and spinal cord. When

Jimm visited, I would tell him how I couldn't study, how stupid I was. He would stand behind my chair and rub my temples in small circles. "Don't think, just study," he entreated, over and over again, an admonition I still use when stuck. At night, on the phone, he listened to me rant – sometimes for hours – about how I struggled with my courses. He brought me Ferrero Rocher chocolates and cups of bad cafeteria coffee, and took me for walks. And even though he struggled with his own demons – his mother had been diagnosed with metastatic cancer at the beginning of his second year – he was always there for me.

"There *is* a method to my madness," he told me sometime that spring. "You're worth it." I wasn't so sure of that, but it was nice to hear.

By that time, I had already decided I wanted to be a pediatrician. The fact that it was very difficult to get a pediatric residency spot only spurred me on. I didn't want to treat adults and the elderly – babies and children, no matter how sick, were much cuter and more resilient. Surgery was too mechanical, psychiatry too fluffy. But how to marry pediatrics with biochemistry? What a weird combination – like those diseases that fascinated me.

At some point during that dreadful winter, in an effort to motivate myself, I hand-printed in block letters on an index card: "There are only four spots in SickKids straight pediatrics internship." This was a coveted specialist internship when one began pediatric training straight out of medical school and not a year later, after completing a year of rotating internship. I taped the card over my desk at home so that I would see it every day. Of course, I wanted to learn pediatrics at SickKids – it was the best children's hospital in the country, after all. To ensure I got a residency spot there, I did the only thing I knew – I studied, I crammed. I had no connections at SickKids, so I was going to have high-enough marks that they – whoever "they" were – would not deny me. I would do my damnedest to get one of those four internship spots.

Unfortunately, I repeated the same mistakes I had made at the beginning of university: I didn't admit to anybody that I wanted to specialize in pediatrics, never asked advice from anyone and did not ask for help. I learned much later, too late in fact, that certain electives with certain staff physicians in certain pediatric subspecialties carried much more weight than others on residency applications.

For the entire second half of the semester, I felt like I was constantly sprinting. If I caught up, I soon found myself lagging behind again. I was exhausted. It was terrifying not to be in control of my studies, my marks and my life, to sense my hard-won future slipping through my fingers. Once, Jimm asked what would I want if I could do anything in the world.

"I'd like to go to a sanatorium," I answered without hesitation. Like those tubercular souls in *The Magic Mountain*, I wanted to have nothing to do, nothing to worry about – no exams, no marks, no studying. I simply wanted to rest and have somebody look after me. Warm myself in the bright Alpine sun, bundled against the bite of the cold in thick woollen blankets, stretched on a deck chair, hot cocoa brought to me by an attentive nurse. Read novels. Sleep in each morning, nap in the afternoons.

I finished my first year without glory, but I didn't fail any courses. Jimm marvelled at how I managed to pull off the marks that I did. During his first year, he had spent so much time trying to learn physiology that he'd failed his neuroanatomy final and had to sit a makeup exam at the end of his summer. Very few medical students dropped out over the four-year course – maybe one or two in every class. Almost nobody repeated a year. My physiology mark, a C, was my lowest of the entire year, but somehow I managed to learn enough to get Bs in pharmacology and neuroanatomy, and passed my elective and the interviewing skills course. My first year of medical school was finally done. I did not flunk out. Looking back, I probably was nowhere near the bottom of the class, but at the time I could almost smell my failure.

3.

The summer after my first year of medical school, I got a research job analyzing the results of a project two second-years had started the year before at Bloorview Children's Hospital in North York. I had applied for the medical school summer studentship to support me, but I didn't get it. My supervisor, Dr. Raymond Tervo, used his own research funding to pay me; the year before, two medical students received funding for the same project – it was enough to make my paranoia return. But in spite of that, I enjoyed drawing conclusions from lists of numbers, finding links and ideas buried in heaps and lists of data. My research examined communication problems experienced by children with physical and intellectual disabilities, and finding ways to alleviate their disabilities with keyboards and desktop computers. There were no iPads in the 1980s.

Bloorview was a two-storey, fully accessible hospital overlooking a verdant ravine just north of Sheppard Avenue. The facility cared mainly for children and young adults with cerebral palsy and spina bifida, many of whom lived there, but infants and children with other neurological conditions were hospitalized there as well. Among the data I was analyzing that summer, I found three children with a rare neurological condition called dystonia musculorum deformans, a progressive and uncontrollable posturing of the arms and legs that rendered their extremities essentially useless. I read all I could about it in textbooks and rehabilitation journals, and proposed that I write a report on the technologies these children used to communicate, such as adapted typewriters and computer keyboards.

Only five years earlier, I couldn't articulate a simple answer on a grade eleven chemistry test, and here I was proposing to write a scientific paper – incredible. I also wrote an article summarizing my summer research, and by the end of the summer, Dr. Tervo had submitted both for publication. A year and a half later, the journal *Pediatric Neurology* released

"Rehabilitation of Communication Impairment in Dystonia Musculorum Deformans," by E. Shahar, M. Nowaczyk and R. Tervo – my first scientific publication. I revelled in seeing my name in print and knowing that it would stay there forever.

But it never occurred to me that I could become a writer of the non-medical type.

✒

One lunch hour in the medical library at Bloorview, I discovered the first edition of Hans Wiedemann's *Atlas of Clinical Syndromes: A Visual Aid to Diagnosis for Clinicians and Practicing Physicians*, and, heart pounding behind my sternum, spent the afternoon staring at black-and-white photographs of misshapen skulls, hands without fingers, genitals that appeared neither male nor female. As I looked at a photo of a squat young man in his underpants, his legs disproportionately short and thick, flesh bunched up above his knees and elbows as if in fetal life his skin had grown several sizes too large for his skeleton, I remembered with a start the untidily cut photograph plates from my mother's *Little Encyclopedia of Health*.

The Wiedemann *Atlas* held pages and pages of photos such as the ones my mother had excised. In the beginning, as I lifted each new leaf, my throat clotted, my heart rate doubled; however, these physical sensations diminished and curiosity won out as I continued to flip through the pages. Upper lips cleft into three fleshy nubbins, pulled up to reveal misaligned teeth and the nasal cavity, did not bother me anymore, nor did lobster-claw hands and clubbed feet. A frisson shuddered through me when I encountered a cloverleaf skull with eyes extruding from their too-small orbits, but even that sensation passed after viewing the photo several times. As exposure desensitization quieted my discomfort, my curiosity deepened – I wanted to know more about the biological processes that led to those malformations, to know how normal development was altered to result in these conditions. And I wanted to know them all. It was almost as if I needed to know how bad, how awful things could get while a person remains alive and human.

No matter how disturbing they were at first, these photographs didn't haunt my dreams. They were only images of diseases collected for the edification of doctors and nurses so that they could take better care of their patients. I had seen photographs of patients in other medical textbooks – endocrinology or genetics – where they were the norm. These photos weren't different from the anatomical drawings in my atlases or the colour photographs of dissections I had studied in my first year – they existed for educational purposes, and were not something to get perturbed about. In fact, the sooner I got over my discomfort, my disquiet, the better. A doctor or scientist had to be dispassionate, professional and detached. If I was bothered by such images, I wouldn't be able to look after actual patients. So, I didn't think about the people in the photos; I only paid attention to the physical findings the images were intended to illustrate.

☞

That summer, without my noticing, my second funny spell ran its course. I was busy collating data, writing two articles and learning how to use a word processor on those early personal computers. I hit the ground running at the beginning of my second year of medical school. I was raring to go, my lassitude and despair gone and forgotten. I hadn't yet learned my lesson – I had not connected this spell to the one I'd had in grade thirteen. In fact, when I saw my psychiatrist that past February, I didn't even tell him about how I had dragged during grade thirteen and my first undergraduate year – I didn't think it was relevant. Both times, I thought what I'd experienced had been self-imposed and therefore deserved: if I only had the moral fibre, the discipline to study, to put my nose to the grindstone, none of that silliness would have happened. Instead, I had indulged in laziness and idleness, and got the bad marks that I deserved.

There was no point crying over spilled milk. Get up, shape up and keep going, I told myself. The only way was forward.

Now that the focus of our studies had switched to clinical courses, the lecturers warned us about "medical student syndrome": the tendency for novice physicians to think they are experiencing the symptoms of the diseases they are studying. Some even saw the signs. I had my share of it, of course: a sharp pain in my left wrist made me think I had lupus; every breast lump was cancer, as was the bony protuberance I palpated on my left humerus, which I later learned was the thickening where the deltoid muscle inserted on the bone; every upset stomach meant I had Crohn's disease.

Of course, this was all in my head – I was healthy as a horse.

One morning during a microbiology lecture on childhood viral infections, the professor mentioned subacute sclerosing panencephalitis – an extremely rare complication of measles that caused a child to lose all intellectual abilities and control of the body. One day, the child would be seemingly recovering from a bout of measles, the next she would have difficulty walking and getting out of bed, soon to become mute and deaf and blind. I'd had measles as a child – there was no vaccine against it back in the '60s. I remember a bright, angry rash on my face when I was four and my mother held me in front of the bathroom mirror.

One day, my grade two teacher sent me home with yet another note for my mother detailing my constant wriggling and insubordination, and asking too many questions in class. That night, I read in the *Little Encyclopedia of Health* about a terrible disease that kids get after measles: "The onset is insidious. Initially there are behavioural changes and the child becomes unsettled, undisciplined, disobedient, excitable or with labile mood. Parents and teachers do not understand the child's illness and administer unwarranted punishment, unaware that the child is ill."[1]

I ran to my mother and told her that this must be the reason I misbehaved in school all the time. "My meanie teacher will be sooooo sorry when she hears about it," I announced. My mother only laughed. "You don't have a disease," she said. "You're just a wicked little girl."

Fifteen years later, in that microbiology lecture, the mention of post-measles subacute sclerosing panencephalitis brought back the memory. I chuckled. I'd had medical student syndrome in grade two.

---

1   Translation mine.

In second year, the courses ran the whole year. The heaviest-weighted was pathology – similar to histology, but the microscope slides bore diseased instead of healthy tissues. The other two were microbiology and pharmacology. We also had two clinical courses, cardiology and respirology, and a half-course titled Alcohol and Drug Dependence. It was in genetics – all about strange conditions that occurred rarely and were difficult to diagnose – where I experienced my epiphany. Most genetic conditions affected children. Many were biochemical. Genetics even had a subspecialty called metabolic genetics – the study and management of biochemical disorders caused by enzyme deficiencies – that seemed tailored for me.

I had found my destiny among the labyrinthine biochemical reactions of the human body.

The genetics course director, Huntington Willard III, PhD, was disliked by most of the class and actively hated by the rest because he demanded that on our assignments and exams we explain the genetic concepts we were learning in grade six–level English. "Pretend you are talking to a patient sitting across your desk," he said.

I grasped the method behind his madness right away. "People hear about pneumonia or heart attacks, but hardly anybody knows about enzymes and genes," I said during an intense discussion about his teaching methods. "I think it's brilliant. Patients need to understand genetic concepts if they are affected by them."

Indignant glares shut me up. "He's not even an MD!" a classmate said, voicing the general consensus. "What does he know?"

It is damned hard to learn the chemical composition and the 3D structure of the double helix, not to mention the laws that rule human inheritance, but having to explain them in layman's terms took the exercise to a whole new level – we had to unlearn the scientific language that set us apart, and in the process learn a new one. Writing "each strand of the original DNA molecule serves as a 5'-to-3' template for the synthesis of its complementary strand and follows the original sequence in a semi-conservative fashion" demonstrated a grasp of the material to our peers and teachers but would be gibberish to most patients. Explaining the genetic code by comparing DNA to a library, with chromosomes as bookcases, genes as chapters in books and mutations as spelling mistakes, required so many more words on an exam that I often had to ask for extra booklets for my answers. At the time, I did not realize that explaining in plain English the mechanics and laws of heredity was what geneticists did every day.

As part of the course, clinicians and researchers gave lectures on genetic diseases they were researching. Ron Worton, whose team was about to discover the gene that caused Duchenne muscular dystrophy, was one of them. I sat there, listening, marvelling at the conditions in which the tiniest change in a microscopic molecule, a single letter alteration in the genetic code, would wreak havoc on a body, perhaps destroy it before it could fully develop. At the time, boys with Duchenne muscular dystrophy died by the end of their teens, perhaps in their early twenties if they were lucky. I thought about the one extra chromosome, the smallest of all them to boot, that caused Down syndrome. That such seemingly minor changes, when multiplied by trillions of cells in the body, resulted in severe diseases highlighted the inviolability of the genetic code. Wouldn't it be wonderful, I thought, if you could just get into every cell and rewrite that one letter of the genetic code or pluck out that extra chromosome and cure patients? Yet, as I enjoyed the intellectual paradox of nanoscopic changes resulting in deadly disease on a human scale, the magnitude of genetic diseases' unfairness astounded me.

After his lecture, I ran down the steps of the lecture hall to ask Dr. Worton whether I could sign up for an elective rotation with him. Or possibly a summer research project.

"I'm not a clinician," he said, "but you should call Joe Clarke." Dr. Joe Clarke turned out to be a metabolic diseases specialist at the Hospital for Sick Children, not the former prime minister of Canada, and my future mentor.

✒

My second, much more painful revelation occurred in the Alcohol and Drug Dependence course: I realized that my father was an alcoholic. When

Monika had blithely announced the same thing a few years earlier, likely as a result of a health class in high school, my indignation had known no bounds. What did she know, the spoiled brat; she had no idea what an alcoholic was. Yes, our father would come home slightly wobbly sometimes after a night out with his buddies, but his choice of drink was beer. Alcoholics drank vodka or moonshine. Dirty, smelly, unshaven men propped the walls of the beer kiosks all over Poland. They were men who wove their way on the sidewalk, staggered home in broad daylight. Men who urinated in playground sandboxes. My father was not one of them.

To me, he only appeared drunk once, and that was when we still lived in Poland. I was nine and he had received a huge bonus at work. Late in the evening, when he still hadn't returned home, my mother phoned for a taxi and left me with three-month-old Monika. Two hours later, the key clicked in the front door and my mother barged in, tossing her purse on the hallway cabinet. My father followed her a bit unsteadily, grinning sheepishly.

"I'm sick and tired of having to drag you from your drinking buddies," she snapped and slammed the door shut behind him.

"Hey, look." He slurred his words a bit. "Here." He thrust his hand into his coat pocket and pulled out a narrow tape of white paper with numbers on it. He waved it in front of her face, wobbling with the movement. "Look at it – the highest wages this month in the entire company. Of everybody. Including the director!"

"I don't care about your stupid pay stub!" My mother snatched the paper and tore it to shreds, threw it in his face. "You think you're such a hotshot!"

It all went blank after that: screaming, shouting, my father's coddled and beloved tropical plants shredded by the windmill of his arms. He didn't lay a hand on us, but I think my mother might have pummelled on his back as he methodically lifted plates from the kitchen cabinets and smashed them on the linoleum floor.

The following morning, I was embarrassed to walk out of our apartment: I was sure that everybody in our building, even those up on the third floor or higher, had heard the screams and noise. That afternoon, when I returned from school, the most awful word from my childhood spread its wings blackly from my mother's mouth: "divorce." She'd had enough, she was getting a law-yer; she deserved a better life, she told her father – she'd phoned him and he'd come for a visit. My grandfather nodded as he rocked my sister in his lap.

I couldn't imagine life without my father. When I was little, I seldom saw him on weeknights – he worked late tutoring university students in math for extra cash – but when he was home we would huddle on my bed and he would read to me. *Winnie-the-Pooh* was our favourite. He showed me photo albums of the Polish archaeological missions in Egypt, and promised that we would travel there to see the pyramids and the ancient temples and the pharaoh's monuments after I passed my baccalaureate exam at the end of high school. "And we'll see the Parthenon in Athens. And Delphi." I knew about the Parthenon, the temple of Athena, the goddess of wisdom and patroness of the Greek capital, and about the Delphic oracle – Greek myths were also on our nighttime reading list; I couldn't wait to see them in real life. When I started school, he taught me algebra and set theory in addition to regular grade one arithmetic.

In Poland, divorce was an unthinkable blemish, a taboo. Even mentioning the possibility of it to my classmates would have tainted me. I sobbed in my locker at school, my nose snotty and leaking. For several weeks, my father hand-dried the dishes and cutlery after dinners, hung new shelves and light fixtures, and nursed back to health the plants that he'd almost destroyed. My mother watched him in haughty silence and held onto her threats.

"When we met, your father would complain to me about his father's and brother's drinking," she told me. "He said he would never be like them. I should've known better."

Five years later, when my mother didn't want to emigrate, she relented only when he promised her that he would stop drinking. And he did, for a few weeks in Austria. But by the time we were living in our new apartment in Toronto, boxes of Molson Canadian began to appear in our kitchen. My father had discovered that venerable Ontario institution, the Beer Store. Preoccupied with my studies and problems, I studiously ignored the empties stacked in twenty-four-bottle boxes in the corner of the kitchen and my parents' fights about them. I escaped the constant tension in the apartment by going to the library to study.

For years, I had managed to avoid the truth about my father, but by the time I was taking the Alcohol and Drug Dependence course in second year, I could fool myself no longer – my father fit all of the criteria of the CAGE questionnaire, a screening test for problem drinking and potential alcohol complications: "Have you ever tried to Cut down your drinking? Are you Annoyed by public criticism of your drinking? Have you ever felt Guilty about your drinking? Have you ever used a drink as an Eye-opener?"

From a lecture on liver disease, I realized with horror that my father's morning retching, which I heard through the thin walls of our apartment, was a sign of liver damage. I was aghast – by then I knew about the complications of liver failure and what awaited him if he continued to drink at his current rate. Every time I brought the subject up, he told me – very Annoyed – to worry about my studying, not about him. I pretended everything was all right even though I agonized over the state of his liver – that it was already failing, that he would die soon. I feared I would never see his blue eyes beam with pride when I became a doctor.

➡

The rest of second year passed smoothly. I studied as well as in undergrad, just as well as I had in the first half of my first year. My marks improved, again, and my future shone brightly. I pointedly ignored what had happened to me the previous year – surely it was an aberration, a blip. I had it licked now. It was probably because Robert had broken up with me. Anyway, I thought, depression was treatable if I really needed it, but obviously I didn't – I had stopped the amitriptyline and got better anyway. And I wasn't really depressed, just worried and upset about my marks, nothing more. I hadn't been very pleasant to be around, that was true, but you'd be unpleasant, too, if you were failing at school. Now that I was studying and not slacking off, I was going to be fine. I just needed to work harder. Jimm made sure I studied, and I enjoyed his attention and the time we spent together.

I had found some companions as well, an eclectic group of students who worked in the empty rooms of the Medical Sciences Building at night, each in a separate classroom: a balding American expat, a recent Vietnamese immigrant and a girl from Quebec. A camaraderie evolved as together we reviewed pathology slides and compared notes. Before exams, we booked study rooms in the Science and Medicine Library's basement audiovisual department, and spent hours flashing pathology slides on the screen and shouting out diagnoses. We actually enjoyed ourselves. Well, I did.

☛

I finished the year with good marks and even managed to get a small scholarship. Things were going to work out – there would be no more laziness and indolence. No more funny spells, I was certain of it.

The summer after finishing my second year I worked with Dr. Joe Clarke at the Hospital for Sick Children. He was the national specialist in lysosomal storage diseases, disorders caused by various missing enzymes that normally turned over cellular components. In storage diseases, the cells and, with time, whole organs ballooned, choked with molecular wastes, and stopped working. Of these, Hurler syndrome was the most severe. I first heard about it back in a first-year biochemistry tutorial when a teaching assistant had told us that children with it would be the ugliest-looking kids we would ever see. "I see them all the time in the Elm Wing at SickKids, somebody there has a clinic for them," she added. How could she say that, I thought? Patients weren't ugly; they have a disease and should be treated with compassion. Especially little children.

That summer, I pored over inches-thick hospital charts, blowing the dust off their covers in the Health Records room on the ground floor of the hospital. Seventeen patients with Hurler syndrome and Hunter, Morquio and Sanfilippo syndromes – related storage disorders – had been treated at SickKids over the previous three decades. The manila folders for several of these charts bore a crimson DECEASED stamp. Dr. Clarke arranged for the patients to come to the clinic so that I could meet and examine them, and update their course in the chart. Even back then, I knew that I was learning from their illnesses, from their misfortune, from their parents' genetic mischance.

Amélie was a three-year-old girl with Hurler syndrome. She reclined deaf, mute and diapered, her head strapped to the back of her wheelchair. Her head was too large for her body – in her brain, the mucopolysaccharide storage had caused hydrocephalus, the "waterhead" of my childhood nightmares. Her thickened lips were not large enough to cover her swollen purple gums or her enlarged tongue. The joint capsules of her hands had thickened and contracted into claw-like appendages. Her abdomen, full of liver and spleen and lymph nodes, filled her lap. I met her knowing there was no cure for Hurler syndrome. For about ten months, Amélie did what all normal children did as they developed – rolled, sat, reached for toys – but then she stopped babbling and cooing, and then stopped sitting on her own. Soon, she wasn't able to hold her head upright. There was no cure for her – she was going to die from complications in her early teens. Bone marrow transplantation trials – an experimental therapy for storage diseases – were just beginning, but Amélie was too old and her disease too far advanced for a transplant.

I imagined myself as Amélie's mother, witnessing that decline, watching her baby daughter deteriorate without any hope of treatment, and decided that neurodegenerative conditions were the worst possible nightmare that a parent could face. This previously normal baby girl, a happy, smiling infant, didn't recognize her mother and father anymore, and had lapsed into a stony silence after only a few months of infant sounds. My imagination failed me and I sat there, stunned. Such destruction because of one spelling change in the millions of letters of the genetic code was beyond my comprehension. And I was scared, sitting in that room, watching Amélie – scared by the inhuman, unyielding ruthlessness of genetic changes that wrecked such havoc on an innocent body. It could've been me, sitting in the wheelchair.

I shook myself and shut down my feelings. I wanted to study these conditions, crack open their malevolent secrets with research, not collapse into a quivering, crying heap.

"We'll need photos," Dr. Clarke said to Amélie's mother when he finished his exam. He pulled a fountain pen from the pocket of his lab coat and slid a stack of small yellow slips across the scratched plastic of the desk. In the windowless clinic room on the main floor of the Hospital for Sick

Children, under the fluorescent lights, this lemon-yellow paper glowed. Line drawings of a person in both front and profile views were printed on each slip. With his gold-tipped pen, Dr. Clarke drew black ovals around the little man's head, hands and feet, and, with a much larger oval, the whole body. He also marked the head and the whole body on the profile view then wrote Amélie's name and birthdate in the upper right corner. His handwriting was even and angular, slanted to the right, and he wrote the date with periods between the numbers, not slashes. I still do it that way myself, thirty years later.

These yellow slips were requisitions for clinical photography: Amélie's physical features and appearance had to be documented wholly and in detail. I thought it was brilliant – no need for lengthy descriptions, just a quick glance at the photo and one knew all one needed to know about the patient's appearance.

"The audiovisual department's on the eighth floor. Take the Elm elevators," Dr. Clarke said, referring to the twelve-storey research wing of the hospital.

"I know where it is," Amélie's mother said and tucked back the white ribbon that held her daughter's thick, coarse hair off her forehead. Dr. Clarke had ordered photographs after every semi-annual visit. The day before, in preparation for the clinic, I had reviewed Amélie's hospital chart: Dr. Clarke had ordered photographs of Amélie the day he'd diagnosed her. In those, the five-month-old already carried the angular peak of a gibbus in her spine (visible on the profile view of her back), showed thickened fingers (close-ups of her hands) and looked at the world with the blues of her eyes clouded (close-up of her eyes). I realized that clinical photography was part of her medical care – it documented the relentless progression of Amelie's disease. I also realized that the photos in the atlases and textbooks I had been studying had to have been shot somewhere, sometime. In the genetics clinic that morning, I witnessed an agreement, an unwritten pact between physician and patient – or parent in this case – that made those photos possible.

❧

The first medical photographs were taken by Dr. Hugh Welch Diamond in the mid-nineteenth century. As the medical superintendent of the

Surrey County Asylum, he began documenting the facial characteristics of patients with mental disorders in 1852 and exhibited his efforts at the Exposition Universelle in Paris in 1855. In France, the eminent neurologist Guillaume-Benjamin-Amand Duchenne was the first to photograph the sequence of movements that a boy with muscular dystrophy had to perform just to rise from lying on the floor; he published them in 1861 in his *Album de photographies pathologiques*. It is the first photographic documentation of a genetic condition.

Photography gained more widespread use in the documentation of skin diseases and lesions, which were frequently hand-tinted to render them more realistically; in the documentation of neurologic and psychiatric disease; and, with the advent of portable cameras in the mid-twentieth century, of surgical techniques. Up until the middle of the twentieth century, medical photographs included images of genetic conditions such as ichthyosis, billed as "fish-baby," or various types of dwarfism labelled as pixies, fairies or leprechauns. Although the practice of such naming has long been frowned upon, those photos still linger in old textbooks.

But in the field of genetic syndrome diagnosis, the face is of primary interest. "Dysmorphology" – a term coined by the father of North American clinical genetics, David W. Smith – is the study of the minor differences of the face that, together, result in one's recognizable appearance. The human eye notices subliminally, instinctively, the minute changes to the shape of one's eyes or chin; the minor deviations from normal dimensions – the length or width of a nose or mouth, the placement of a hairline or eyebrows on the forehead. We perceive these as "different" or "dysmorphic," as we do with changes in the shapes of pupils or nostrils; an extra row of eyelashes or the presence of dimples in an unusual position on one's cheek.

Anthropometry – the measurements of distances on the face and head such as between the corners of the eyes or the length of the ears, and circumferences of the skull taken at various landmarks – is used extensively in plastic and reconstructive surgery, but in genetics, a syndrome diagnosis is frequently made by inspection alone. Photography is the easiest and most logical way to record such features, and it is much more expeditious than words. In medical genetics "a picture is worth a thousand words," if not more. In his 1866 paper, John Langdon Down did not publish photographs of the syndrome that would bear his name; he relied on medical language instead:

> The face is flat and broad, and destitute of prominence. The cheeks are roundish, and extended laterally. The eyes are obliquely placed, and the internal canthi more than normally distant from one another. The palpebral fissure is very narrow. The forehead is wrinkled transversely from the constant assistance which the levatores palpebrarum derive from the occipito-frontalis muscle in the opening of the eyes. The lips are large and thick with transverse fissures. The tongue is long, thick, and is much roughened. The nose is small. The skin has a slight dirty yellowish tinge, and is deficient in elasticity, giving the appearance of being too large for the body.[2]

That so many words are needed to describe a facial appearance that we all recognize in the blink of an eye makes photography an obvious choice for the documentation of facial features.

Our medical textbooks were full of photographs of patients. When a photo showed the whole body, the patient's eyes were blacked out with rectangles, giving them a raccoon look, but in the documentation of syndromes, blacking out the eyes would defeat the purpose of photographing the face in the first place. The area around the eyes provides too many important clues to syndrome diagnosis: the length and shape of the eye opening, the arch of the eyebrows, the clue-rich area between the inner corners of the eyes – the nasal root and the glabella – the smooth part of the forehead between the eyebrows. Extreme close-ups of these structures couldn't be used, either – geneticists needed to see the whole, the gestalt, not its parts at a remove.

---

2   J. Langdon H. Down, "Observations on an Ethnic Classification of Idiots," in *Clinical Lectures and Reports by the Medical and Surgical Staff of the London Hospital*, vol. 3 (London: John Churchill and Sons, 1866), 259–62.

The first photographs taken specifically of dysmorphic features were published in 1911 in Charles Davenport's controversial and now reviled treatise, *Heredity in Relation to Eugenics*. Davenport commented on subtle heritable "minor anomalies" – upturned noses and receding chins – in a grandmother, her son and granddaughter as illustrated in the photographs of their profiles. At the time, eugenics journals also published photographs of traits, including facial appearances, while genetics journals began publishing such photographs in the mid-twentieth century.

Eugenics was increasingly discredited as unscientific and racially biased during the twentieth century, especially after its doctrines were adopted by the Nazis in order to justify their treatment of Jews, disabled people and other minority groups. Modern human genetics – the study of human variation and inheritance of biological traits – has divorced itself vehemently and completely from those horrors committed, erroneously, in the name of science.

When David W. Smith's *Recognizable Patterns of Human Malformation* appeared in 1970, it became an instant classic; there is no clinical geneticist in North America, and probably the whole world, who has not studied its black-and-white photographs in detail. By now, many colour plates have replaced its original images, although the rarest of rare conditions are still illustrated by the black-and-white photos of earlier editions. Since the penultimate edition – its seventh – an online version also exists.

✒

One day, near the beginning of that summer, I sat hunched over a radiology textbook in a carrel in the SickKids' medical library, writing down the skeletal anomalies observed in mucopolysaccharide storage diseases. When bone cells are distorted by the lumpen storage vesicles, the bones growing around them become misshapen, too. In the early days of radiology, physicians let their imaginations run wild with metaphors to better describe the shadows of organs and bones on black films. And since radiologists never had to deal with patients, some of these were quite odd. "Bullet-shaped phalanges" – the tiny bones of the fingers and toes; "beaking" of the front aspects of the vertebrae; "paddle-shaped" clavicles and ribs. That day, as I was busy acquiring a whole new vocabulary and an appreciation for medical humour, a soft tap landed on my left shoulder. I turned to see a man I had never seen before – a beaming, relaxed Jimm. His shoulders were not propping up his ears; he stood straightened and tall, his handsome mouth stretched in a grin from ear to ear.

He'd been so morose that spring, so worried about his third-year comprehensive exams that I had seriously considered breaking up with him. His mood had been dark enough to eclipse the sun; his conviction that he would not pass into clerkship was strong enough to engulf me in its spinning vortex. Fortunately, I was doing well enough that year to sustain both of us.

"I passed!" he whispered into my ear – strict silence was observed in medical libraries back then. I giggled – his breath had tickled me.

And just like that, I fell in love with this happy, carefree man.

✒

As I reviewed the clinical notes on old patients with Hurler syndrome, I noticed that three had congenital glaucoma: they were born with increased fluid pressure inside their eyeballs, probably caused by the glut of storage material in the conjunctiva, the tissue that cushions the eyeball in the socket and lines the inside of the eyelids. I checked in the genetic and biochemical textbooks and in papers on storage disorders, and I couldn't find any previous mention of this complication. Dr. Clarke agreed that it was worthwhile to publish. My second paper, "Glaucoma as an Early Complication of Hurler's Disease," published in the *Archives of Disease in Childhood* in 1988, is still quoted in genetics textbooks and on the more obscure reaches of the Internet.

✒

"Anybody in the hospital who can interpret in Polish, please call 7500." The voice overhead pierced my concentration. On a late Sunday afternoon in July, I was reviewing the charts for the next morning's clinic in the fellows' room, where I had a desk for the duration of the summer.

Polish! I couldn't pick up the phone fast enough. Finally, my mother tongue would be an asset rather than a hindrance.

The paging operator took down my number and said they would call me.

The phone didn't ring until two hours later. By then my excitement was all but gone – I was hungry and wanted to go home.

"The resident will meet you on 4B," the operator said.

The resident explained that she needed to obtain consent for the insertion of a central intravenous line, a catheter threaded directly into the superior vena cava, the large vein that delivers blood to the heart. It would allow doctors to administer drugs and to sample blood for tests without repeated needle sticks – I didn't realize at the time that the drugs would be chemotherapy. When we entered the room, a little girl was huddled against her mother's breasts, arms around her neck, big blue eyes pools of shadow. She was very blonde and very scared.

"I don't speak any English," her mother said in Polish after I introduced myself. "She has cancer atop her kidney and they need to start chemo. I don't understand anything." She looked down at her daughter. "She's only three years old. Children don't get cancer!" Unspoken in her eyes was the perennial question: "Why my child?"

The resident rushed through the explanations. I did not understand how she could be so callous – couldn't she see the mother's fear and confusion? I struggled to keep up under the torrent of words, realizing then that I did not know Polish medical terminology. A translator's job only looks easy. I muddled through my explanations as best I could. The mother signed the consent form and the harried resident left the room.

"Co myszko?" I asked the little girl. She ducked her head under her mother's arm like the little mouse I just called her. I also did not know any terms of endearment in Polish, and that hurt even more than my limited Polish medical vocabulary. The latter could be easily fixed, but I had missed out on the former too long ago – my mother was more likely to call me an imp and mean it.

Before leaving, I wished the mother all the best. Wilms tumour was curable with a great success rate. The little mousie would be fine.

On Monday, I asked Ron, the hematology fellow who shared an office with me, about the little girl.

"Wilms tumour? We have no new Wilms," he said, furrowing his brow. "Last night we admitted a girl with neuroblastoma – stage four."

Although I knew nothing about neuroblastoma, "stage four" told me enough. It usually denoted incurable cancer – the tumour had metastasized to distant sites.

It hit me.

"I ... I thought it was Wilms," I said, shocked. "The mom said 'on top of her kidney.'"

"Yeah. In the adrenal," Ron said, compassion shining in his eyes. I felt so stupid – to have felt hopeful, to have wished the mother all the best when the mousie's prognosis was so dismal.

Before the end of the summer, I stopped by a few times to check up on the little girl. The last time I visited, she sat alone at a small easel in the playroom tracing pink wiggles on the dusty blackboard using chalky fingers. She smiled shyly, cocking her head like a little bird when I spoke to her in Polish, but she never answered. With each visit, she became more and more pale, the defenceless pink of her scalp peeking between thin blonde strands as her hair fell out.

A week later, I started my third year of medical school. I never learned what happened to the little mousie, but I thought about her frequently. I didn't check up on her because I was not in her circle of care and felt that I shouldn't. And maybe because I was scared of what I would find out.

☛

In third year, all of the courses were clinical: endocrinology, ophthalmology, psychiatry, obstetrics and gynaecology, surgery. And finally: pediatrics. I had not made a mistake in my choice of specialty – when I studied child development or the differences between adult and children's diseases, the knowledge, the information just flowed into my brain and stuck in my cortex without any effort. I loved everything about it: the challenges of examining wriggling children, the way growth and development altered the physical presentation of illnesses, the long lists of diseases that infants and children could develop. "What's the difference between adult medicine and pediatrics? Adults get four diseases that present in a hundred ways, children get hundreds of diseases that present four ways." The four ways were vomiting, crying, not eating and not playing.

I also enjoyed the lectures on psychiatry. I did not see myself at all in the descriptions of patients with depression. But I found psychosis and personality disorders fascinating if a bit scary and felt for people with obsessive-compulsive disorder: How could they function, lead a normal life? The challenge of navigating daily life with a psychiatric condition that intruded all the time captivated my imagination: How could one get any work done if for every time they read the word "pencil" they had to perform some kind of ritual? Or if they had to wash their hands five times after every time they touched a doorknob?

That November, after a lecture on mood disorders, it occurred to me that it would be nice to be hypomanic: full of energy, needing little sleep, goal-oriented and non-distractible, with heightened perception, an iron will and a sense of purpose. According to our psychiatry notes "increased energy, expansiveness, risk-taking and fluency of thought associated with hypomania can result in highly productive periods." What a contrast to the hopelessness, anhedonia and lassitude of depression. Of course, I wouldn't want to be manic – the psychotic high of bipolar disorder is where judgment fails completely. But hypomania was the way to go, especially before exams. How well I could study then! How well I would do on my exams! Just a bit of hypomania, I joked, would suit me very well.

My medical student syndrome failed me completely: I *was* being hypomanic. I thought I was just being me – the me I loved being: exuberant, happy, achieving. They didn't teach us this part in the psychiatry lectures – patients with mood disorders lack insight into their condition, especially when in a midst of an episode of depression or mania. Or maybe the teachers had mentioned it, and I – lacking insight – didn't register it.

As before, I studied by writing and rewriting lecture notes and whole paragraphs from textbooks. In my green, hardcover study notebook, I detailed case histories of patients from the hospital clinics, and hand-printed pages of notes on their conditions copied from the two-volume *Harrison's Principles of Internal Medicine*, and from recent articles I looked up in specialist journals. Whenever I got an answer wrong, whenever I misunderstood a concept, I scribbled my old friend PAŁA on the margins of the notebook. I was still constantly marking myself, hoping that shame would goad me to work harder, to get better marks. Years later, a psychologist treating me asked to see those notebooks and his eyes goggled at the sight of the PAŁAs marching along the pages after I had explained to him their meaning. The notebook is also full of "loving" admonitions, all in capitals: "I AM SORRY BUT YOUR ORGANIZATION OF THE CLINICAL EXAM LEAVES A LOT TO BE DESIRED!!! YOU BITCH!" or "DON'T BE TOO COCKY!!! DON'T MAKE SPOT DIAGNOSES! YOU DO NOT KNOW ENOUGH."

"Just look at this," my psychologist said. "These notes demonstrate an in-depth grasp of medical concepts only a fraction of people on this planet can understand, and yet you thought that you were stupid." I shrugged – I *was* stupid if I couldn't remember the significance of the "a" and "v" waves of the jugular venous pressure, or the seven types of glomerulonephritis.

He asked my permission to photocopy several pages of the notebook as an example of obsessive-compulsive tendencies – my minuscule and copious handwriting, my demonstrated self-loathing, my squadrons of PAŁAs admonishing me. "I will only say that you are a high-achieving academic," he said. I said yes.

☛

Jimm's mother died in October of my third year of medical school, his fourth. She had been diagnosed with metastatic breast cancer when he was in second year, shortly before we met. After her death, the powers that be allowed him only three days' leave from his pediatric clerkship to arrange and attend her funeral – there was actually a kerfuffle about his on-call schedule. As stubborn and shy as he is, it never occurred to him to ask for help. He used the nights on call and constant studying as balm for his heartbreak and, unlike me, seldom complained. Instead, he worried himself sick that he wasn't studying enough and that he would fail his exams. I tried my best to support the man I loved, but soon I wasn't able to do so anymore.

The last note in my green clinical medicine notebook is dated February 2, 1988. By that time, I languished in the library every afternoon trying to study, but knowledge refused to enter my skull, medical facts bouncing off my cortex. Fear ate at my innards – the comprehensives loomed on the horizon; in around three and a half months I would have to sit the final, three-day-long exams, covering all the subjects we had studied since September, and pass two clinical oral exams. I was freaking out – there was no way I would pass any of the subjects if I did not start studying immediately.

Once, on a group project, I told the supervisor that I would do my best on it. He replied that everybody in my clinic group would do their best.

"Well," I said. "I assure you that I will."

He repeated, sounding irritated: "You *all* will do your best."

"I can't speak for others, can I?" I think he was trying to teach me teamwork, but how could I guarantee anything but my own performance? I wholly believed that I couldn't speak for the others' work ethics. He shook his head unhappily.

The winter days dragged on. I had no contact with my clinic-mates outside of school. We did not study together; we did not discuss our progress. I didn't admit to anybody that I wasn't studying, that I couldn't concentrate; that I sat for hours staring blankly at open textbooks and notes. I was sure that they would only take advantage of my weaknesses, leave me behind in the dust. Show me up in clinics. Belittle me.

✒

Every time my depression lifted, I believed it was my last episode. Just a blip. That first time, back in high school, I had no idea what was happening. The second time, it had a name and a treatment, and I believed that it could be treated, would be treated, and that I would be fine from then on if I continued therapy. When it hit again, and it hit hard, I panicked. I did not dare admit to anybody but Jimm that I needed help. Like a fish tangled in a net, I flailed about with my notes and textbooks, overwhelmed by the amount of material I had to study. I showed off when I did know an answer. I snapped at the slightest provocation like a stepped-on snake. I would apologize, but the damage was already done – people started to avoid me.

When finally I didn't show up to hospital clinics – one skipped clinics only if one was on one's deathbed – and went to the dean's office asking for help, a woman from my clinic group noticed me waiting there. She came in not to ask how I was but to tell me how much I had upset the whole clinic group with my behaviour. Unsaid, but implied, was that I should be more considerate of their feelings. I didn't know what to say in my defence.

"Are you coming back?" she asked at last.

"I don't know." I really did not know if I would return to clinics, to studying, to medical school. At that moment, dejected, slumped on the waiting room chair, I did not think myself capable. But how could I quit medical school? Not after everything I had done to get in.

I didn't quit then. I returned to clinics and tried my best to study. I did reasonably well on the written exams but bombed on the clinical oral exam. Much too late, I learned that others practised in teams to deliver cases quickly and efficiently, learning to be organized and succinct. I did not practise for the final clinical oral exams at all – I didn't know how to do it without asking for help. During the exam, I could not list even a fraction of a cogent differential diagnosis for a patient's congestive heart failure, and did not outline proper investigations and requisite medications. I stammered. I backtracked. The cardiologist who was marking me looked livid. He minced no words – I was disorganized and unprepared. He gave me a C. Yet a week earlier, on a practice oral exam with another clinician, I had done really well. That examiner had even complimented me on remembering that pregnancy might have deleterious effects on a patient with congenital heart disease. What went wrong?

John, a classmate from another clinic group, sat beaming in the lounge when I shambled in with my C. We had met earlier that afternoon when the supervisor handed us the names of the patients assigned to us for the exam.

"How did it go?" he asked.

"I totally messed up." I was almost crying.

"I had a physician for my patient!" he announced gleefully. "He told me his entire history, all his meds, and even reminded me of the common side effects of digitalis! Told me what type of heart murmur he had!"

He had aced his oral. My first thought was that a physician should not have been a patient for a clinical oral exam. My second, that I could've gotten the helpful doctor if only the exam supervisor had switched the cards.

I dragged myself up Bathurst Street and east on Harbord Street to the haven of Robarts Library. I broke down and sobbed, crumpled in a concrete staircase linking the book stacks. I bemoaned the scholarships and awards that I would never get, the pediatric residency at SickKids that would never accept me. Jimm found me there an hour later but even he couldn't calm me down. He had finished his clerkship rotations and was to graduate from medical school the next month, relieved that his ordeal was over. If I'd had any insight, any idea of how unwell I had been, I would have been happy that I managed to pass the year. Without it, I could only sit and cry.

☛

Two weeks later, morose and unhappy, I began my fourth year – the clinical clerkship portion of medical training at St. Michael's Hospital in downtown Toronto. That year, we would pass through four- or eight-week rotations in surgery, internal medicine, pediatrics, psychiatry, family medicine, and obstetrics and gynaecology, as well as two-week rotations in anaesthesia and ear, nose and throat surgery. There were also three four-week elective periods to explore personal areas of interest – pediatrics for me.

My first rotation was family practice. I tried to overcompensate for my failures, both real and imaginary. Once, I took so long to examine a patient who had a simple cold that her boyfriend complained to the receptionist, worried that something had happened to her. My evaluations, deservedly, stank. During my next rotation, psychiatry, I hijacked a one-on-one teaching session to present a litany of my own problems and worries. I think I was hoping for some understanding, maybe even help. The psychiatrist sat there, impassive, and listened attentively, I thought. Later, he wrote on my evaluation that I was "unable to separate personal concerns from clinical ones." Feeling utterly betrayed, I promised myself never again to speak to anybody about my problems.

I really wasn't doing well at all but I didn't know it yet.

Beginning in mid-August, I started my eight-week elective block. I had arranged for a rotation in pediatric neurology and another in general pediatrics at the Izaak Walton Killam Hospital in Halifax, the pediatric referral centre for the Maritimes. On the overnight eastbound train – I took a train because I wanted to see more of Canada and I had heard that the Atlantic provinces were absolutely beautiful – I tried to forget my poor showing on the first two rotations, tried to talk myself up to the task, to show that I deserved to become a pediatrician. Elective rotations, ostensibly for exploring new areas, were really intended for impressing supervisors so that they would write glowing reference letters for internship and residency applications. I had to do well if I wanted to have a glimmer of hope of ever getting into SickKids.

But my depression followed me like a bad stink. I ticked off my Haligonian peers. I annoyed my supervisors. It was only then, when I performed poorly in the rotations I cared so much about, that it dawned on me: If I was to have any future in medicine, I couldn't, shouldn't, go on. I was hurting myself and those around me. I needed to stop. Even before I returned to Toronto, I placed a long-distance phone call to the Student Affairs Office and made an appointment with the dean of Student Affairs.

The last Monday of September, I boarded the Toronto-bound plane in the pre-morning darkness at Halifax Stanfield International Airport. After landing at Pearson, I took a taxi directly to school and explained the situation to Dean Ross Fleming. He listened quietly, nodding as if in understanding, but he would not guarantee me a place in next year's fourth-year class if I took the year off. "If nobody fails their third-year exams, there won't be room for you in clerkship," he said. "Are you sure you want to stop?"

I was not so far gone that I didn't care about not having a position when I was ready to return, but I also knew that I had to get out.

"I can't go on," I said.

He stared at me for a moment then unscrewed his fountain pen. "I'm not going to put 'mental health issues' as the reason for your leave of absence," he said. "I'll just put 'medical problem.'" Such was the stigma associated with mental illness that I was genuinely relieved. I thanked him.

4.

Imagine taking an indefinite, precarious leave of absence from the only thing in life that matters to you. Imagine turning away from what you have fought for years to achieve, throwing away dreams and hours and days and years of studying and cramming and sacrificing.

Walking away from the present of medical school meant jeopardizing the only future I thought I had. If there were no vacancies on the student roster the following year, I would have nothing to show for eight years of post-secondary education. What if I never got back in?

My plan was simple: I would take time off and, with the help of a psychiatrist, uncrumple the pages of my life. A psychologist did not factor in – their services were not covered by OHIP and I couldn't afford to pay out of pocket. I figured that therapy wasn't going to take too much time so I decided to also audit two Russian literature courses at the University of Toronto and practise my French in a conversational class at the School of Continuing Studies. I'd had enough of science and medicine for now.

Good plan, except that I could not find a psychiatrist. My old psychiatrist wouldn't see me – probably because I stopped seeing him against his advice back in my second year of medical school, when I was doing so well that I thought I would never need his help again. None of the others I approached had openings to take on a new patient. One who did insisted that I start psychoanalysis, which was too scary and too time-consuming a prospect. Another intimated that therapy would take at least a year or two "because that's how long a personality change takes." I told him that I liked my personality well enough and did not wish to change it. And I didn't want to wait years for results – I needed help now.

Someone recommended a woman psychiatrist who had recently opened a private practice in the imposing sandstone Medical Arts Building on the corner of Bloor and St. George. When I phoned her, she explained that she could only provide a consultation, that she had no openings for long-term therapy patients. I was so miserable and scared that I went to see her anyway, hoping that she would take me on for pity's sake or out of professional courtesy. For an hour she listened to my life story – my worries, woes, dreams and fears. Then she told me that I had clinical depression, that I definitely needed therapy and that it would likely take a long time for me to get better. But no, she did not have any therapy spots available, and no, she didn't know anybody to refer me to. Then she asked for my health card number. I had forgotten my OHIP card and promised I would call her with it as soon as I got home.

I slunk out of her waiting room, ducked into the stairwell next to her office, slumped on the top step and burst into tears. I didn't care if she could hear me. I don't remember how long I languished there before I trudged the six flights down to Bloor Street.

I did not call her with my insurance number that day – my French class was in the evening and I did not get home until late. The next morning, my mother woke me up at 8:00 a.m. with the phone in her hand – it was the psychiatrist.

"If I don't submit the claim by the end of the month, I will not get paid," she said.

"We can both see what's important to you, then, can't we," I hissed. I didn't care what she thought of me. She wasn't taking me on as a patient and I didn't have to be meek. I rummaged around on my desk for the card and read the number to her before I slammed the phone down.

Another psychiatrist, who treated me briefly during that time, sent me to a psychiatric specialist at Mount Sinai Hospital for a second opinion without telling me why. The consultant – a soft-spoken, bespectacled man in his sixties with a nice, soothing voice – talked to me for an hour. At the end of the consultation, he said that I had a good, strong core and that I would "be all right." When I checked the papers and books he had published, to my dismay they all focused on personality disorders.

So that's what they all thought: I had a personality disorder, the condition nobody wanted to deal with. Not depression or psychosis or obsessive-compulsive disorder but a personality disorder – the anathema of psychiatry, intractable and untreatable. In our psychiatry clinics, we had been taught that such patients were wholly unlikeable – inflexible, maladaptive, incapable of meaningful long-term relationships, lacking in empathy; they made frequent, unconvincing suicide attempts as a means of manipulating those around them. They were impulsive and moody. Was that who I was? I wracked my brain to figure out which of the telling medical school mnemonics for personality disorder clusters I belonged to. Was it schizoid, schizoaffective, paranoid? No way. Was it avoidant, dependent, obsessive-compulsive? Maybe? Or was it the rest: Borderline, narcissistic, antisocial, histrionic? I couldn't be borderline, could I? That most dreaded of personality disorders? After all, I had a devoted boyfriend, I did not cut myself and I had never attempted suicide. I had empathy for my patients. I was not a sociopath.

After all that, the psychiatrist who had requested the consultation with the personality disorders specialist had his secretary call me at home to cancel my next appointment. He never offered me another.

➡

In the end, it was Jimm who found a psychiatrist for me – a woman who was "interested in issues of women in medicine." He heard about her from a psychiatrist at Toronto General Hospital, where he was doing his internship. I phoned her and she agreed to take me on as a patient. Dr. Margaret Whitfield turned out to be supportive and kind. Every Wednesday afternoon I rode the subway to the refuge of her office on the ground floor of a modern house on a tree-lined street in Toronto's Chaplin Estates. I don't remember the details of what we talked about, but for the first time in my life I felt that a woman listened to me without passing judgment.

In late November, when I started psychotherapy with Dr. Whitfield, I also began to plan my return to medical school. I didn't want to fall out of the habit of studying, of being a medical student; my intention was always to return when I felt better.

Because I loved pediatrics so much, and because I thought it would rekindle my love of medicine, I arranged to shadow Dr. Katy Driver, a staff pediatrician at SickKids. At ten in the morning on Tuesdays and Thursdays,

I would meet her in her downtown office at Central Hospital. Housed in a four-storey building, the hospital was founded by two Hungarian-Jewish physicians – the brothers Paul and John Rekai – in the early 1950s, and since then it had established itself as the primary hospital serving the immigrant population of downtown Toronto. It was also an entry point into the Canadian medical system for immigrant physicians who were waiting to qualify in Canada. Jimm's father, only the second Greek physician in Toronto, had worked there since he arrived in Canada in 1953. George, my ex-boyfriend, had folded bedsheets in the hospital laundry during his first summer in Toronto, and Jimm had been a gopher in the hospital laboratory for several summers. He remembered collecting blood and urine samples from Dr. Driver's office.

"You're going to love her," he told me. "She has a whole wall of kids' photos in her office."

He was right – I did love working with Dr. Driver. She was a petite South Asian woman with kind brown eyes that seemed to be always smiling. She was apprised of my situation by the Dean's Office and took me on without any fuss. She never even mentioned it – I wanted to be a pediatrician and she was happy to show me the ropes.

By ten in the morning, her windowless, tiny, sparse waiting room would be already full of patients: sleepy newborns for their first post-delivery checkup, cooing infants, toddlers holding onto chairs taking wobbly steps as they waited for their vaccinations and sullen teenagers who really didn't want to be there. Dr. Driver's no-nonsense approach rubbed off on me mothers were always right about their children, babies didn't need to be babied. Patients were examined and prescriptions written out with a smile and wink. She never addressed parents as "Mom" and "Dad," a habit I abhor.

She admired babies, but not too much, and stuck vaccination needles into arms and legs without much fuss. She taught me how to examine a toddler in a mother's lap, to make them more cooperative; how to get a scared child to open their mouth and say "ahhh"; how to find the light reflex on the eardrum; and how to pinch the skin on an infant's chubby thigh for an intramuscular injection of a diphtheria-polio-tetanus vaccine.

I listened to tiny lungs whooshing and hearts beating at twice the rate of an adult's; learned how to recognize a yeast diaper rash and what ointment to prescribe for it, and how to differentiate between the rash of fifth disease and that of hand-foot-and-mouth disease. Once, she admonished a young mother against putting her son to sleep with a milk bottle – the toddler's teeth were brown and rotten to the gums. I think I learned most, if not all, of my primary pediatrics in her two-room, bare-bones office on the third floor of the medical building on Sherbourne Street.

Over the lunch hour, Dr. Driver drove her gold Mercedes sedan to SickKids where she was one of the two physicians working for SCAN: Suspected Child Abuse and Neglect. That was also part of pediatrics – recognizing the signs of non-accidental injury and abuse prevention. It had turned my stomach to learn, during our third-year pediatrics lectures, that there existed parents who hurt their infants and toddlers on purpose. I could not comprehend it: How could a person hurt something so helpless, so trusting, so vulnerable? Twist tiny arms or legs until they cracked, squeeze so hard their ribs snapped, shake their tiny bodies until they bled in their brains? At first, I didn't think that I could handle going with Dr. Driver on SCAN rounds, but she made it if not understandable then at least bearable. The team's goal was to protect the child and that I could relate to.

After rounds at SickKids, we were often late for Dr. Driver's afternoon clinic in her second office at Don Mills and Lawrence. There I met children from some of the poshest mansions in Toronto – the Bridle Path and Post Road were just around the corner from her office building – to whom Dr. Driver extended the same no-nonsense attitude, advice and medical care. But it was a world apart from what I saw at her downtown office.

One afternoon, a china doll–like four-year-old girl was brought in for an asthma flare-up by her nanny and her teenage half-sister. Dr. Driver asked me to examine the girl as she lay sprawled in her sister's lap.

I stuck my stethoscope in my ears. "Wanna take your blouse off?" I asked the girl. Telling young children to undress themselves usually worked like a charm – most loved shedding their clothes at the slightest suggestion.

The girl stared at me with pellucid blue eyes that appeared ... disdainful?

What the heck?

"She can't do that," her sister said, and the nanny nodded. The girl just lay there, motionless.

Oh my god, I thought in horror. The girl's paralyzed, she has some terrible neurodegenerative disease or something, and here I asked her to do something.

"She never does anything," the sister continued, lifting the girl's arms and pulling the sweater off over her curly mop. "Irene does everything for her." Irene, the nanny, bent down to unfastens the girl's shoes. Dr. Driver didn't bat an eye as she placed the bell of her stethoscope on the girl's chest and listened to her breathing.

Not paralyzed. A princess.

Between Dr. Whitfield's support and therapy, and Dr. Driver's non-judgmental attitude, the confusing, strange and scary irritability, hopelessness and fear I felt ran their course. I thought mine was an isolated situation, but what I was going through was not, and still isn't, that uncommon: over the past thirty years, more than a quarter of medical trainees reported experiencing either full-blown clinical depression or depressive traits during their training. Burnout and anxiety were common, but the self-imposed isolation and shame prevented me from reaching out to others who might have shared my predicament.

By spring, I was ready to return to medical school. In spite of Dean Fleming's concerns, there was a spot open for me in the incoming clerkship year. As luck would have it, the sequence of rotations I was assigned began with pediatrics, which was fantastic – I couldn't wait to show how much I had learned working alongside Dr. Driver. However, my home base was Toronto General Hospital, which was not so fantastic.

All medical students knew that "the General," the flagship of Toronto's Faculty of Medicine, was the toughest hospital for clerkship and internship. But I had no choice. My standards had dropped from the stratosphere of ambition with which I had started medical school. But I still wanted to graduate with honours; I had ever since seeing the honours graduates lead the convocation procession at Jimm's graduation that past June.

By the last week of September 1989, in addition to pediatrics, I had gone through the clerkship rotations of obstetrics and gynaecology; ear, nose and throat; and anaesthesia services, and had done very well. For the long-houred rotations – obstetrics and gynaecology, internal medicine and surgery – I had moved into a room in the Toronto General Hospital residence, another brutalist, beige-grey concrete bunker across Elizabeth Street from the hospital. I had loved my four-week-long pediatrics rotation and received a ninety. Not gold medalist material, but definitely honours. During every rotation, I had arrived early and stayed late, done everything I was told to do and then some. But internal medicine, the eight-week rotation I was just about to start, had the reputation of being the most brutal of the whole year.

"I was the gold medalist in my medical school class, you know?" the ward chief said the first morning of the rotation. I cracked a smile just as I realized he was dead serious. Myopic eyes drilled into me, pale blue beads behind thick lenses. He wore an impeccable, starched white coat, his name embroidered on the chest pocket. He steepled his thick fingers as he crossed his legs. The lines of power were clearly drawn and crackled, electric – he was a world-renowned internal medicine specialist, while I one of six clinical clerks starting a rotation in internal medicine. An observation I'd heard as a medical student about the hierarchy of a teaching hospital was that "on top is the ward chief, then the consultants, then the residents, then the interns, then the nurses, then the janitor, then the dirt on the floor and *then* the clinical clerks." It would have been a great joke if the comparison wasn't so apt.

This ward chief's reputation preceded him. "He marks people down. He's brutal," Jimm told me in response to my theory that a gold medalist should make for an easy marker. Who but a medalist would understand the desire for good marks? "Forget it," Jimm said. Not fair, I had thought. Why begrudge a few marks if you've already arrived?

And there he was: my supervising attending for the next four weeks – and the ward chief, as he reminded us.

☞

On my first night on call, a thirteen-hour shift that started at 5:00 p.m., the senior resident and I were responsible for all internal medicine admissions. My first patient of the evening was Mr. B., a tall, gangly Hindu man with chills and a fever. His wife had died of AIDS a year earlier, in Uganda; infected himself, he lived with his brother in a northern suburb of Toronto. His brown eyes burned in his emaciated face. His lips were dry and bleeding, the insides of his cheeks pitted with shallow grey craters. Pity coupled with revulsion and fear flooded through me: What if I contracted AIDS from him? At the time, AIDS was still a deadly and uncurable disease.

"He's yours," the senior said. "Full infectious workup." Read: detailed medical history, a complete physical including a rectal exam, blood work. An hour later, he reviewed my admission notes and, without changing anything, scribbled his name under mine. I had been complimented on my clinical notes by several staff physicians – pertinent negatives and pertinent positives in order of importance, a list of active problems in order of significance, each with an appropriate treatment plan. I wrote the admission orders for the senior to co-sign before the nurses could carry them out.

Back in Mr. B.'s room, I watched the nurse start an IV in his forearm. What if she stuck herself? I held my breath as she carefully inserted the intravenous cannula and dark blood flowed back – lethal, full of virus. Finished, she dropped the used needle into the bright yellow stay-away sharps container.

My first internal medicine admission, done, and countless more to come.

☞

I startled out of dreamless sleep on a hard bed in a darkened room. I lay there as if at the bottom of a black well. Tall buildings listed toward me, casting shadows across a flimsy, threadbare curtain drawn partially across the window. The crisp smell of hospital laundry. A piercing noise battered my eardrums. Where was I? Where was here? My heartbeat thumped in my belly. I checked the time. I had gone to bed forty minutes earlier, around 2:00 a.m. I turned off the hysterical pager and sat up. The number flashing on the green screen didn't register in my mind, but I dialled it, my hands shaking.

"This is 10E." I wasn't on call for ward 10E. "Mr. H. on your ward has just had a run of vee-tach."

"A run of what?" I could hear my voice shake.

"A patient on your floor who is on cardiac telemetry has just had a run of a potentially fatal arrhythmia," the nurse enunciated.

"What am I supposed to do about it?"

"You're the doctor," the nurse said and hung up. I stared at the phone. A jumbled list of antiarrhythmic drugs from first-year pharmacology flashed in my mind, illuminating only fear. I wasn't allowed to give intravenous medications. I needed help. But I knew that calling the ward senior for something that a clerk is supposed to be able to handle was evaluation suicide. Was this one of those things? I decided that "useless" branded on my forehead was better than "dangerous." I dialled the senior's pager and waited.

"There's a man with vee-tach on my ward," I said when he called back.

"Have you examined him? Done an EKG?" he fumed.

History and physical! Of course, I remembered, but absurdly, history and physical were not going to fix this patient's problem. I needed to know what to do about a "potentially lethal arrhythmia." I slouched off to the nurses' station – I had been sleeping down the hall in a patient room converted to an on-call room. My surgical greens were too big for me – my pants trailed along the floor. My white coat was weighted down by manuals, drug compendia, tuning forks, ophthalmoscope, stethoscope. My yellow nametag hung askew on my breast pocket, where my ID picture showed somebody who looked like me but ten years younger.

I found the patient asleep in his bed, alive and well. When I woke him, his pulse raced to a hundred beats per minute. His blood pressure was normal, and he grumbled when I hooked him up to the EKG machine.

By the time the senior arrived on the ward, he had cooled off. He reviewed the EKG strip, pointing out the abnormally shaped wave complexes that were popping up at irregular intervals, like speed bumps on a city street, and explained that the team would reassess him in the morning. He even taught me a few things.

☛

The next Saturday, my day off, the phone in my dorm room rang. It was 5:35 a.m.

"Tato's going to the hospital," my mother said. "He woke up with that burning in his chest again."

For weeks, I had been trying to get my father to see Dr. Abramowicz. "I'm not your patient," he'd retort. "It's not angina – it's just my skin." He had rubbed his hand in a small circle just to the left of his sternum, not the typical clenched-fist-to-the-chest Levine's sign of a heart attack that all students know by the second week of medical school. He had fooled me.

Jimm stirred next to me. He had spent the night and was on call again today, starting at 8:00 a.m., back in London, Ontario.

"My dad's going to the ER. Chest pain." My own heart beat a crazy staccato in my chest and my mind rolled ahead: my father was having a heart attack, he was going to die, he would not see me graduate. If I had stayed in school last year, I would have been a doctor by now.

As Jimm sped uptown along the empty morning streets, I told him about my grandmother's fatal heart attack at the age of sixty-one. We lived on the other side of Poland at the time, and my father took the first available train and still did not make it in time to see her. At her funeral, my cousin Renata howled at the graveside, my blind grandfather called for his babcinka little grandmother – as my father watched, stone-faced.

When we arrived at North York General Hospital, I jumped out of the car. The ER doors whooshed open to reveal my father sitting at the triage desk. Alive. I stifled a sob. "My skin is burning, here," I heard him say.

I rolled my eyes. "It's chest pain," I said to the nurse. "He's had it for weeks."

Even with chest pain, he didn't let my mother drive him to the hospital. His racing pulse and his appearance – wan and tremulous – got him onto a stretcher in the central bay of the emergency ward and hooked up to a heart monitor within minutes. "I'll get the EKG machine," the nurse had said as she rushed out. My father's face glistened with sweat, his skin ashen. His eyes shone like blue alarm beacons.

The EKG squiggles were unmistakable. Deep waves flooded the pink millimetre graph paper, threatening to overturn the tiny boat of my father's heart. A plaque had exploded and blocked his left coronary artery, and his heart flailed like a fish out of water, gasping for oxygen. I stared at the EKG, the line flipped from normal, showing small currents fluttering in an undertow. If I could only reach into his chest, push through skin and muscle and ribs, scrape the vessels clean with my fingernails, I could fix it before the damage was irreversible.

I tore the sheet from the machine and dashed to the physician sitting at the main desk. "My dad's having a heart attack. Why isn't somebody doing something about it?"

He looked up from the charts in front of him – a big, soft teddy bear of a man, kind brown eyes filling his thick glasses – and barked, "And who are you?"

"I'm a medical student. Just look at this, please. It's my dad."

The teddy bear glanced at the printout and got up. He knew that there was only so much time to make a difference.

My father lay propped on the bed, hooked to an IV, oxygen prongs on his nose – the panic in his eyes gave him the appearance of a beached walrus. The nurse had a syringe ready.

"Three milligrams morphine," the teddy bear said. My father cracked a tiny smile, summoning all his charm to wriggle out of this one.

"I don't need all this, Doctor. My daughter exaggerates. It's not angina. It's my skin," my father said, his English rough, with short vowels and a hard "g" barely audible over the hiss of the oxygen.

"You're having a heart attack." The authority in the teddy bear's voice stopped all arguments. "I'm getting the cardiologist to get you some medicine to dissolve the clot." Fear replaced the pleading in my father's eyes.

The cardiologist arrived within the hour and I learned more about streptomycin in five minutes of talking to him than I had learned in a year of cardiology lectures. My father said he understood the risks of stroke and of bleeding into the brain; I did not. The infusion was started within the required time, but only just. My father admitted that pain had woken him up at four in the morning and that he had thought a hot shower might take it away. When that hadn't worked, he had taken another. Disloyalty sitting heavy on my chest, I told the cardiologist about my father's drinking. They started him on Valium to prevent delirium tremens – the dreaded DTs – the potentially fatal consequences of abrupt withdrawal from alcohol.

My mother arrived with my sister. I wanted to have a good cry on her shoulder, but she was hysterical. I needed to be strong for her. My sister watched us both, her eyes the same blue as my father's.

☛

"Fifty-eight-year-old woman admitted with a two-day history of dizziness." The senior, the interns and the ward chief stood guard around the wheeled cart loaded with patient charts as I presented the previous night's admissions. Eight patients had blurred into a many-headed hydra waving a laundry list of signs and symptoms. "She has a past history of cer– cerebellar– celeberral latelar stroke." After eight years in Canada, I still struggled with pronouncing r's and l's when they came in pairs or in sequence. I mangled "palarreroglam," "celebral." Throw in a w, "jewellery," and my speech became a fiery plane crash, ideas smouldering at my feet.

"La-te-ral ce-re-bel-lar stroke," the ward chief enunciated. "I thought it took a certain level of intelligence to get into medical school."

The senior resident smirked. With English as my second language, I've always relied on the intelligence of strangers, I wanted to say, but I stopped in time. They probably wouldn't get my *A Streetcar Named Desire* reference anyway.

☛

The next day I approached the ward chief after morning rounds.

"My father's having a cardiac catheterization at the Western. I'd like to be with him. He had a heart attack two weeks ago ..."

"I know. What are you going to do there? This, here, is your work. When my son was five and being investigated for meningitis, do you know where I was?" His eyes narrowed. "Right here."

My eyes goggled – I've died and gone to *The House of God*.

By the time the rotation was half done, I had lost five pounds. I lived in my surgical greens and had stopped wearing makeup. My father's angiogram had shown a left ventricular aneurysm, which meant he had a poor prognosis for recovery, as Dr. Waye, a kindly consultant cardiologist I cornered on the ward one day, explained to me. After, I stared out the hallway window for a long time, wondering whether my father would live long enough to see me become a doctor.

The senior emerged out of the clean utility room. "You want to know your mark?" he asked in a low voice.

"Yes." A steel fist clutched my stomach. I hated getting my marks.

"The staff met at lunch today. You did okay. With your dad and all. Mid-seventy or so."

There had been a time when I would have considered this a failure.

"Thanks. He's home now." My father had come home the day before, his pants hanging loosely from his belt, cheeks pink again under the purple stain of fatigue that surrounded his eyes. He had hardly spoken in the car and had gone straight to his bedroom when we got back to the apartment.

The senior stared at me for a moment, his forehead wrinkled in confusion. "Oh, you mean your father," he said and marched away.

"You asked the senior to give you your evaluation?" The ward chief cornered me by the elevator later that same day, his voice quiet yet menacing. "I give the evaluations here."

"He came up to me this morning and offered ..."

"That's not what he said."

I opened my mouth but stopped myself. There was no point. This mark was only a third of my evaluation. A new attending and a new senior resident were starting the coming Monday. I could still do it. I could still get honours – mathematically speaking.

☛

I went home that evening. It meant a long commute at six the next morning, but I wanted to spend as much time with my father as I could.

"Don't worry so much," he said, as I washed the dishes after dinner. "I'll be okay. I'm so proud of you."

He's just saying that, I thought. "I did not do so well on the first part of this rotation," I said. "I got a B. Not honours."

"What is 'honours'?" he asked.

"Marks above eighty. Like a 5? I want to graduate with honours."

"Why?" He sounded genuinely puzzled.

What kind of question was that? I wanted honours because I wanted to show my worth, to show that I could succeed in spite of my mispronunciations and my last name. He did not know how important marks were when dozens of candidates from around the world applied for eight pediatric residency positions. Yes, eight, not four like I thought during my first year of medical school.

My father had grown up on a small farm in Lasek, a hamlet south of Poznań, surrounded by four loud and boisterous older sisters. His brother, the eldest and eighteen years my father's senior, had married and moved out by the time my father was born. Three other sisters had died – the second eldest before World War II, from appendicitis at age twelve, and the two born just before and just after him as infants less than a month old. My grandparents were not rich – they owned half of a house, two hectares of land and a garden with a dark, echoey well hidden in the corner behind gooseberry bushes. Their barn held a single horse, a cow, two goats, several pigs and assorted poultry. His mother tended the house and the livestock; she grew vegetables that she sold at the Jeżyce farmers' market in Poznań every Thursday. His father worked at the Singer potato starch factory in Luboń, a neighbouring town. My father grew up kind and happy. In a favourite photograph I have of him from his childhood, he stands next to one of his sisters in front of my grandparents' house. His face is split in a toothy grin under a goofy hat with earflaps. His jacket and pants are shabby, many-times mended. I loved that smile the moment I saw the photo – an exact replica of my older son's smile.

In his one-room village school in the late 1940s, my father was always the first to solve any math question the teacher wrote on the blackboard. At lunchtime, he built hydro turbines using potato halves and matchsticks, and ran them in the stream bordering the schoolyard. After finishing public school in grade seven, he attended a three-year trade school and qualified as a die cast operator, but he wanted more. He got a job at the village post office delivering mail and enrolled in night school. When I visited Lasek with him as a teenager, neighbours regaled us with tales of my father leaning on gateposts, book in hand, solving algebraic equations as he waited to hand over the mail. Once or twice a month, he boarded a creaky local train to Poznań that puffed steam out its smokestack, and attended symphony concerts and the opera. He always read on the train. Once, enchanted by the Polish national epic *Pan Tadeusz*, a nineteenth-century twelve-book poem set in alexandrine verse, he missed his stop and had to trek back home along the rails through the midnight darkness. All Polish schoolchildren were required to memorize its invocation – my father memorized the entire first book. When, for his sixty-fifth birthday, I handed him a two-volume first edition from 1834 that I had managed to buy from a Polish antiquarian, he had tears in his eyes.

After obtaining his baccalaureate, he wrote the entrance exams for the engineering faculty at the Polytechnic Institute in Gliwice. Based on his score, he received a full scholarship for meals and a room in the dormitories; there were no tuition fees in Communist Poland's universities.

Once there, he spent his nights playing bridge and chess, and beating his roommate at a guerrilla memory game they had invented: at all times of the day, they would challenge each other to define words from the *Dictionary of Foreign-Origin Words*; at the end of each month, they'd tally up points and the loser had to buy dinner. And yet he still managed to excel at his studies. My parents were married at Christmas in 1963, his last year of university, and he defended his master's thesis six months before I was born in December 1964.

"You've always been so ambitious," he said to me that evening over a frothy sink full of greasy pans, my hands reddened from the hot water and detergent. "From grade one, you'd cry if you didn't get a 5. You don't need it anymore, you know?"

He did not know how important marks were when your clinical supervisors weren't your parents' friends. He didn't know about my well-connected med school classmates who had not arrived in Canada with fifty dollars in the unfathomable emptiness of their fathers' wallets and who drove their own Porsches to hospital clinics. He didn't know how much marks mattered when you had nothing.

How could I explain it to him?

Lois, the new senior resident, was earnest and competent. She laughed easily, a clear, tinkling laugh so different from the sycophantic cackling of my previous senior. She knew exactly what went on: "He purposely loses to the cardiology attending at squash every Tuesday morning."

"What's this, a sewing circle?" the ward chief asked when he saw us together for the first time. The three of us – Lois, Joan (the new intern and my former classmate) and I – were the only all-female internal medicine team in the hospital. Although not on service anymore, the ward chief popped up on the ward, a liege surveying his domain. One rainy and blustery November afternoon, he entered the nurses' station where Lois and I were writing notes in patient charts. Lois had just finished doing a spinal tap, and her long brown ponytail was still tucked away under the collar of her white coat. He sidled behind her and reached to either side of her neck, looping his fingers under the hair and slowly pulling it from her coat. Lois's back went rigid. Her pen stopped moving across the page.

"Better?" He patted her on the shoulder. After he left, Lois gaped at me, her silence screaming.

One morning, Mr. B.'s brother approached me in the hallway and handed me a note. "My brother wants you to have this," he said.

I expected a thank-you card, a note of gratitude. I unfolded the paper – writing in Hindi covered the page from edge to edge.

"I cannot read this," I said and smiled.

"It says, 'I just want you to fix my mouth. I came to the hospital because of my mouth. I cannot drink. I cannot swallow. Stop doing all these tests. I do not want them anymore.'" Mr. B.'s brother studied my face as he spoke. I felt my cheeks grow hot. I was the only one who touched Mr. B. I entered his room every morning, checked his pulse and blood pressure. He never spoke to me. I should have thought about his mouth care myself.

I blinked. Why was the brother smiling?

"I will take care of this," I said. I sidestepped around him to the nursing station. I hid in the corner and stared out the window at the first snow-flakes blurring the nearby buildings in the opaque light of the morning.

☞

Lois recommended an idiot-proof on-call manual, a spiral-bound booklet that I studied every evening and carried with me everywhere. I memorized its approaches to common in-patient problems and experienced no more middle-of-the-night panic about arrhythmias or urine retention. This was how I should have studied for my third-year orals, I realized, much too late. With Lois's guidance, I performed spinal taps and arterial stabs, but not on AIDS patients – those Lois did herself. I learned things from her painlessly, by osmosis. My confidence grew. I studied for the rotation exam with the determination of a miner staring down a rock face.

Support also came in the form of a neurologist assigned as my faculty mentor. Dr. Catherine Zahn treated me with respect and humour, and taught me how to perform a brief yet thorough neurological examination. She was a ray of sunshine in the torrential downpour of misery and self-blame and inadequacy. She always asked about my father and reassured me about my abilities. I looked forward to our biweekly sessions as if a dose of sanity in a crazy world.

My final examiners were a nondescript endocrinologist and a general internist with a handlebar moustache and a bunch of keys attached to the belt loops of his tight black jeans. They observed me interview and examine a Latvian grandfather of three with a mop of grey hair and a kind smile. He was older than my father, he had come to the hospital with the first twinge of chest pain and he had no permanent damage to his heart.

"The patient is a seventy-six-year-old male with a recent history of a myocardial infarction admitted for percutaneous balloon angioplasty of the left main coronary artery." My presentation flowed effortlessly. Questions followed: What is the first line of treatment for acute myocardial infarction? Morphine and oxygen all those weeks ago. How do you evaluate cardiac muscle function after a heart attack? An angiogram that I was not allowed to attend. How long is the recovery from a heart attack and how is the patient rehabilitated? Cardiac rehab classes and a bland, low-fat Canadian diet, a readjustment for our whole family. No more bigos with fatty pork swimming in spiced sauerkraut, no more Wiener schnitzels. The examiners threw in some questions on chronic obstructive lung disease and fluid management, and it was over.

"Excellent," said the general internal medicine attending, ticking off boxes on his clipboard. "Eighty-five." The endocrinologist nodded.

I almost skipped back to the ward, where Lois told me that I was reliable, that my knowledge was impressive for a clerk, that she was amazed about how well I had done "considering everything." She gave me a ninety for the second half of the rotation. I calculated quickly and: Yes! I was going have an A in internal medicine!

At 4:00 p.m. that afternoon, I met the ward chief in his office to get my final mark.

"Great mark on the oral," he said as if it were his own accomplishment. "Your final mark is seventy-eight." I had calculated and recalculated my mark since this morning, in my head and with a calculator. He must have lowered my initial ward mark to sixty to get a seventy-eight overall. But it had been a mid-seventy, the senior had said ...

"Anything else?" This time he actually smiled.

And suddenly I just did not care.

☛

The ward hallway stretched dimly in the December dusk. Doors to patient rooms opened on both sides, all of them familiar to me. Mrs. S. relaxed in her bed, back from the surgical ward, her esophagus mending from a rupture during a transesophageal echo; I had made the diagnosis one evening when her neck puffed up. Next to it, the room where Mr. C. stayed before he went for resection of a frontal lobe glioblastoma. When examining him, I'd found that his right leg was so weak that he could not stand straight or walk three steps; the admitting team had never asked him to stand up and my senior was ecstatic that he could show up his counterpart on the other team. The room next to the stairwell was where Mr. B. had died. None of the biopsies, needle pokes and bone marrow aspirates had cured the mouth ulcers that had troubled him so badly.

Lightness filled my chest and limbs. Marks do not matter. I bobbed on the air like a balloon escaping a birthday party. Marks do not matter. I looked down the hallway and my epiphany sparkled in sharp relief: My knowledge and skills were solid. I knew my worth.

The elevator dinged and I got on. I was free.

☛

On the surgical rotation, I spent two weeks each on orthopaedics, neurosurgery, thoracic surgery and general surgery. Rounds kicked off at six every morning, with operating rooms (ORs) starting at eight o'clock sharp. When not assisting in the ORs, I took care of any acute problems facing patients on the wards and took part in consultations for other services in the hospital and in the emergency department. I liked the thoracic surgery fellows the most. They were funny, intelligent, capable – and they spent upward of twelve hours in the hospital every day. Two were American – Harvard graduates, no less – and were here because Toronto General Hospital was a leading training and research centre in lung transplantation. The first time in the operating room, I watched in awe as the crumpled, brown sponge of a collapsed lung that had been deflated for surgery blossomed into pale, pink-petalled flowers. I watched as the tissues closest to the bronchi expanded first and, centrifugally, filled the surrounding tissues. Soon, the pink loaf filled the whole chest cavity. The surgeon stitched the rent in the pleura, the ribs sprung back together from the spreaders and the skin hid the wonders beneath it. That day, I wished I knew how to write poetry.

Neurosurgery rotation followed, which was filled with controlling ego-maniacs, one of whom kicked me out of his operating room three times before finally allowing me near the operating table to hold the retractor. He could tell, he said, that I hadn't scrubbed my hands sufficiently because they were not reddened enough.

Orthopaedics was mainly carpentry. What does it take to be an ortho-pod? Be as strong as an ox and twice as smart. This adage did not do justice to my instructors, who were smart and funny and self-deprecating. Only one, across the street in Mount Sinai, had an ego that wouldn't fit through a barn door. When a student questioned something he had said, he answered, "Because I am a professor and who are you?"

The long winter nights and the early hours wreaked havoc with my sleep. An underground tunnel connected the residence to the main wing of the hospital, one part of the web of long, featureless, drab corridors beneath the downtown hospital core. One night in January, I woke up in the dark, panicked, convinced I was late for morning rounds. Luckily, I had slept in my surgical greens. I rubbed my finger against my teeth in lieu of morning toilette as I pounded the elevator button with my other fist. The elevator discharged me in the basement and I raced down the tunnel toward the hospital. When I emerged from the elevator at the other end – up this time – and ran onto the emergency floor, I glimpsed the clock above the sliding door: eleven thirty. At night. As I processed the positions of the clock's hands, I realized that I had collapsed earlier that evening after finishing work and had woken up only five hours later, my addled brain thinking it was morning. I skulked back to my room.

It was not the first time my internal clock had malfunctioned after a night on call. In August, on the obstetrics rotation, I had crawled back to my room and tumbled into bed at 4:00 p.m. after thirty-four hours spent seeing patients in clinics, and assisting in the OR and delivering babies. When my alarm went off at six thirty, I jumped out of bed, dressed, put on makeup (that was before internal medicine, when I still cared about how I looked) and dashed across the street to the hospital. It had been a beautiful summer morning, even if the light seemed subdued somehow. I did not realize that it shone from a completely wrong quadrant of the sky for it to be morning. When I made it to the eighth floor of the Eaton Wing, I was miffed that the team was not there yet – rounds started at 7:00 a.m. sharp.

"They were here earlier, but they've left," the charge nurse told me.

"But we have rounds at seven!" I was indignant.

"No, you don't," she said. "You were on call yesterday, weren't you?" she asked.

"Yes. No! I was on call the day before, on Tuesday."

"You were on call last night. I was here."

I stared at her.

"It's Wednesday. You went home, slept and came back the same evening," she said as if she had seen it before.

"No, it's Thursday morning," I insisted lamely and looked around.

The ward clerk shook her head. "It's Wednesday evening," she said.

"Why don't you go home and get a good night's sleep?" the charge nurse said.

I did.

☛

Match Day came – the day when medical students across Canada are assigned by a central computer to a year-long internship after finishing medical school. This day would determine my future. In my rankings, I had put the Hospital for Sick Children as my first and only choice for a straight pediatric internship. Other than plastic surgery and ophthalmology, it was probably the most prestigious and difficult-to-get internship position in Toronto, if not the whole country. My other, far, far less appealing choices were rotating, non-specialty internships in several Toronto teaching hospitals.

I picked up my envelope in the Student Affairs Office and, heart thumping in my throat, ripped it open. I had been matched to a rotating internship at Women's College Hospital. For a demented yet blissful moment, I had actually thought that I got my first choice because Women's was my first choice of non-pediatric internships. The bubble of happiness burst the moment I realized that I did not match to the straight pediatric internship.

We had signed a contract when we registered for the matching process – there was no getting out of this. I read my sentence, my banishment, and slinked around the corner, bravely yet barely keeping it together when I heard a colleague say into a nearby pay phone, "I matched to pediatrics at SickKids!" I gaped – he had never uttered a peep about wanting to be a pediatrician. Now crying openly, I darted to the basement of the FitzGerald Building next to our medical school. It had an old-fashioned women's bathroom with a tiny side room featuring a plastic beige chaise longue. I lay there for a good hour, sobbing, inconsolable, until I felt well enough to call Jimm in London. He was all concern and support, but he couldn't fix it either. I went back to the General where, in the hallways and in the residents' lounge, on the wards and in clinics, I would have to face the beaming and the happy, the chosen who'd gotten their first match.

Fortunately, for the time being I was the only clerk assigned to the psychiatry ward – a temporary refuge and my rotation at the time. During my four weeks there, I managed not to compare myself with any of the hospitalized patients. One day, Dr. Richard Swinton, the attending, pointed out a young man with schizophrenia recovering from his first episode of acute psychosis. The man staggered around the ward, emaciated as if he had been physically ill for weeks. Dr. Swinton was a fine man – attentive, sincere and very, very good at what he did. I think he recognized how unhappy I was, yet he always had a smile for me.

"He's the best example that psychiatric diseases are physical," he said. I nodded sagely. Of course they were. Already, I was a firm believer that neurotransmitter imbalances caused psychiatric manifestations and disease.

Several patients whose depression had resisted all known forms of therapy were being treated on a research basis with a brand-new drug called fluoxetine, better known now as Prozac. It was the first of the selective serotonin reuptake inhibitors (SSRIs), a new class of drugs that would soon make a difference to millions of people. One such patient, a previously almost catatonic forty-two-year-old woman, happily announced after a weekend pass that she and her husband had gone dancing for the first time in years.

"They did the 'fluoxtrot,'" Dr. Swinton said wryly during morning handover. He chuckled at his bad joke, but he looked pleased about her progress. It was obvious how much he cared about his patients.

I had four patients assigned to me. I was supposed to meet with them every day and record how they felt, what they thought, if they had any plans for the future. I told myself that I only needed to do one at a time and not worry about the others. And I did. Every morning, I would greet one of "my" patients and invite him or her to join me at the battered table in the common room heavy with cigarette smoke. Occasionally I managed to cajole them out of bed, but sometimes they refused outright. After we chatted, I wrote notes, signed them and moved on to the next patient feeling like I had accomplished something. On and on this went, every morning. I learned that, no matter how unhappy and miserable I was, if I simply put one foot in front of the other, over and over again, I could get things done. I studied my psychiatry notes and textbooks in the evenings in the hospital library. In the end, I did very well on my oral, and Dr. Swinton gave me an A for my ward mark.

I was surprised. "I had such a hard time working this month," I said.

He smiled. "I know," he said. "But you worked hard and you deserve the mark."

☛

The next rotation, family medicine, was rockier, probably because I did not think much of academic family medicine in a tertiary teaching downtown hospital. I couldn't hide my disdain. I don't prevaricate well. But I got a good mark there, too.

And then it was over. I had finished medical school. I was a doctor.

Two years earlier, I had asked a clinical clerk who had just finished his last rotation what it felt like to be done.

"Remember *Full Metal Jacket*? When they leave Vietnam?" he asked. "Like that. Going home."

I had never seen the movie but got the gist of his simile. I laughed. When I finished writing the family medicine exam on the Friday afternoon of the final week of the final rotation of the final year of medical school, I remembered his words.

I was going home. Wherever that was. I had finished med school.

☛

Moments before the graduation ceremony on June 8, 1990, as we donned our academic robes and were handed our ceremony programs, I was delighted to read my name on the honours list. There had been no announcements, and since I didn't get an A in internal medicine, I had thought – obsessively – that my marks would not be enough. I and forty-nine other honours students led the procession across the Front Campus lawn to Convocation Hall, that same lawn I had scanned five years earlier when I had received my medical school acceptance letter. As I took my seat, I saw Jimm waving at me from the balcony opposite. He gave me the thumbs-up: he had figured out from my place in the procession that I'd got what I wanted. That month, he was finishing his first year of residency at Western University in London, Ontario, and was returning to Toronto on July 1 – he had been offered a second-year internal medicine residency position at Mount Sinai Hospital.

In the graduation ceremony program, I read that the chancellor of the university would drape the royal-blue-and-crimson hood over our heads during the ceremony and utter the Latin formula *"Admitto te ad gradum"* – "I admit you to the degree." But when I knelt in front of John Black Aird that afternoon, he grinned and said, "What a great smile," as he draped the hood on my neck. He never uttered the magic words! I was handed my diploma after I stepped from the dais and there I was – now, officially, a doctor of medicine.

The ceremony over, we spilled out onto the grass of the Front Campus – yes, it still smelled of camomile – where my parents and Monika and Jimm waited for me. Earlier, while I had been fussing with the gown and carried the hood folded over my arm to the ceremony, my father had run around the Front Campus photographing every building along King's College Circle. Once we emerged, he'd shot our procession and me in it. He had used up an entire thirty-six-exposure roll of film. "So that you will remember what the university looked like on the day you graduated," he told me. For family photos and photos with Jimm and my professors, he had to load up a new film cartridge.

☛

I began my internship at Women's College Hospital on July 1, 1990; the dreaded July 1 when, on the stroke of midnight, all the doctors-in-training advance a year in their responsibilities and bear the stunned deer-in-headlights look. It's the day when newly minted interns – recent medical school graduates – do not respond to being called "doctor" because it is still so new to them. The new interns joined their medical teams, which consisted of residents – trainees who have finished their internship and were continuing further in training to become specialists.

General surgery was my first internship rotation and I was put on call one-in-two for two weeks, which meant I was on call every other night. The surgical chief resident believed in the "sink or swim" method of learning. I managed well, especially since the other surgical interns and residents were fun to work with.

During the summer, I had applied for a residency position at SickKids as well as several other pediatric training programs across Canada. If I were accepted, I would be at the same level of training as new interns accepted out of medical school, while my original classmates, with whom I'd begun medical school five years earlier, would become my seniors. In early September, I had an interview with Dr. Alan Goldbloom, the SickKids residency training program director. I thought it went well. Now, I could finally think about getting married.

Jimm had proposed on December 31, 1989, my twenty-fifth birthday. My parents were thrilled at the prospect even though they were disappointed that Jimm and I nixed the idea of a big wedding in the bud. We invited twenty-five of our closest relatives and friends, and made reservations for an evening reception. We were getting married in the Roman Catholic Church so we had to participate in premarital classes at a week-long retreat in Mississauga. Arranging that particular weekend off was a nightmare. I had asked for the weekend off three months earlier, as soon as I had signed up for the retreat. To my dismay, the physician in charge put me on the overnight shift on the Friday night, claiming that I still had the weekend off because I was not working Saturday or Sunday! It was in the emergency department at SickKids, during my pediatric rotation, and the last thing that I wanted to do was rock the boat, fearing that I would jeopardize my chances. So, meekly, I attended the Friday evening retreat session after which Jimm drove me back to the city for my overnight shift that began at 8:00 p.m. The following morning, bleary eyed and interestingly pale, I listened to a nun explain the rhythm method of birth control.

Jimm and I were married on October 6, 1990, on a windy but gloriously sunny morning at Saint Augustine Chapel in Scarborough, where the Polish Roman-Catholic parish my parents belonged to was housed at the time. Monika was my maid of honour – the only bridesmaid, actually – and Jimm's brother, Kosta, was our best man. Jimm and I took a "honeyweek" at Millcroft Inn in Alton and at Killarney Lodge in Algonquin Park, and the following Monday, after five wonderful days in the wilderness, hiking and meeting moose and canoeing and chasing loons on the lake, we were both back at work.

At the end of that Monday afternoon, in the locker room as I was getting ready to go home after a full day of work on the internal medicine ward, my pager shrilled. It was Dr. Goldbloom, calling to offer me a residency spot at SickKids for next July.

"Are you still interested?" he asked.

"Of course I'm interested!" I shouted into the phone.

☞

Because I didn't have to prove myself anymore, I relaxed and began to have fun working as a doctor. I was starting intravenous lines in old ladies with no visible veins – a talent I discovered I had that year. I could thread a catheter into a stone if need be. In the emergency room, I learned how to set broken bones and stitch up cuts and gashes. But it wasn't all fun. Once, while on call for internal medicine, I pronounced four people dead in less than twenty-four hours and signed their death certificates with my name. When I crawled back to the call room at six that morning, I could hear through the open windows sparrows rioting in the trees lining Grenville Street; sad and upset, I ached to get out of there, yet I had to wait another two hours for the morning sign-over rounds. In ICU, I stood rooted to the floor as I witnessed a forty-three-year-old woman die from alcoholic liver cirrhosis. Splayed on a waist-high bed as if on an altar, she bled from every orifice and into every body cavity, hooked up to beeping monitors, alarms sounding constantly. We couldn't replace her blood fast enough in spite of the intravenous lines we threaded into her heart and pulmonary arteries. Her panicked eyes flitted between our faces. The brilliant blue of her irises still haunts me.

☞

That winter, during my second surgical rotation, as the world watched Operation Desert Storm, depression slithered back into my life.

I did not care about Desert Storm. I did not care about anything. Luckily, interns didn't have to assist in operating rooms since there were enough residents who had to learn surgical skills, as well as numerous clinical clerks who were marked on attendance. So, after the morning ward rounds, I could easily slip into the lounge on the fifth floor. In the mornings, the lounge was empty – ward rounds on more reasonable services started at 8:00 a.m., while the surgeons were already operating. I lay on the couch and stared at the TV, the volume switched off, the new all-news channel flickering as it had been for the previous two weeks – all Desert Storm all the time. Iraqi missiles heading toward Israel momentarily convinced me that I was witnessing the start of World War III, but even the threat of a nuclear holocaust, delivered in the breathless commentary of the Scud Stud Arthur Kent, failed to rouse me.

One morning, as I lay on that lumpy sofa, a thought popped into my mind: if it could be guaranteed that I would not suffer, I would kill myself. I wanted to simply stop feeling this useless, this worthless. This awful. But there might be a hell, after all, or something worse, and that thought kept me from doing it. But from that moment on, thoughts of death were my constant companions on that couch.

What was I moping about? I had everything I had ever wanted: I was a doctor, I was married to a wonderful man who loved me, I was going to start my training in the field I had always dreamed about and at one of the leading hospitals in the world. Life couldn't be better. The future shone brightly. And yet there I lay, flattened on a shabby sofa in the residents' lounge, stirring only when somebody showed up with a lunch tray and I realized that it was nearing noon. I was not hungry.

By April, this spell too had lifted, without treatment this time. The natural course of uncomplicated and untreated depression is a spontaneous resolution within six to eight months. Luckily, mine did not last that long: on July 1, 1991, I started my pediatric residency at SickKids.

5.

On a sunny Monday, July 1, 1991, just before eight in the morning, the heat of the summer day not yet boiling over, I put my right foot on the rubber mat that activated the door of the Gerrard Street entrance to the Hospital for Sick Children. The glass door whooshed open and I became a pediatric resident at SickKids – my dream came true. I was beyond eager to soak up the knowledge, learn pediatric clinical skills and meet my new colleagues, who I was convinced would become lifelong friends. We couldn't afford not to, such was the reputation of the program: it was tough and demanding, just the thing to build camaraderie and friendships.

It was going to be brilliant.

The Hospital for Sick Children was founded in 1875 and has been on the leading edge of pediatric patient care and research ever since. The Salter pelvic osteotomy to repair congenital dislocation of the hip and the Mustard procedure to correct fatal heart defects in "blue babies" were developed there in the 1960s. In 1968, SickKids opened one of the first neonatal intensive care units in North America, devoted exclusively to the care of critically ill newborns and premature babies, and in the 1980s its research institute became a leading centre for genetics research with the identification of the genes for cystic fibrosis and Duchenne muscular dystrophy. As a place to train as a pediatrician or a pediatric surgeon, a clinical researcher or a scientist, it had no equal in Canada, and very few around the world. And since it was a teaching hospital for the University of Toronto Faculty of Medicine, the hierarchy I experienced so painfully during my clerkship was in full force. Except now I would be a little bit higher on the ladder – a resident.

After a brief orientation that morning in the drab residents' lounge on the eleventh floor of the University Wing (battered sofas, rickety armchairs, a pool table and an enormous rear-projection TV set), Joanne, another first-year, and I crossed University Avenue to Mount Sinai Hospital where we began our neonatology rotation in the seventh-floor neonatal intensive care unit (NICU), a rarefied world of bright artificial lights and hushed voices, where the tiniest of tiny babies sojourned, each suspended in its own temperature- and humidity-controlled incubator. The following eight weeks were a frenetic blur of normal and premature deliveries in the adjacent high-risk pregnancy unit; teaching and work rounds; dictating pages-long discharge summaries on babies that had spent almost as long in the nursery as they had in the womb; and learning, learning, learning, the tedium enlivened by twenty-four-hour shifts every four days that wreaked havoc with our circadian rhythms.

I remember distinctly one night being asked to baptize a dying newborn. She was born on her due date, but she weighed just under a pound, the size of a five-month-old fetus. Her parents had known that the baby wasn't doing well from her first ultrasound eighteen weeks into the pregnancy, but they didn't want any prenatal testing. Other than the child's much-too-small size, the doctors and nurses awaiting the baby had no idea what to expect.

When she arrived in the NICU, it was obvious that there was something really wrong with her. She wasn't just tiny; she also looked different. And while nobody on the neonatal team could put the minuscule eyes, the pointy chin, the skull too large for her teeny body into a recognizable whole, we all knew that she was too tiny and too fragile to survive. After she was placed in the incubator – a tiny exotic fish in her own heated, humidified and oxygenated aquarium, and wrapped in a pink blankie barely a foot square – Jean, the Belgian NICU fellow, left to talk to her parents. They had decided during the pregnancy not to keep the baby alive if she was too sick – they wanted "no heroic measures," but he needed to confirm their wishes now that their daughter had been born. Sometimes, seeing and holding a warm, soft baby that had been only an abstract thought for months changed even the strongest of parental convictions.

When Jean returned from the mother's room, he said, a bit bewildered, that the parents wanted the baby baptized. The nurse and I looked at each other – it was three in the morning, the baby was dying and we were in a Jewish hospital.

"A doctor can do it in such a case," the charge nurse said.

Jean shook his head. I said I would do it.

From behind the main desk, the charge nurse retrieved a book of Christian lay ministry where we read that a physician could indeed baptize a baby, and that the baptism would be recognized by the Catholic Church if an appropriate formula was followed and the baptism eventually reported to the nearest Roman Catholic parish.

The fellow shook his head again. "You can do it, if you want to," he said to me. I did. I wanted to feel like I was doing something for this little mite.

Still incredulous that I was allowed to do this, I lifted the book from the nurse's hands. She had also brought out a black box; when she opened it, I saw a glass vial of holy water and a crucifix. I had been raised Roman Catholic and was prepared to do what the parents had requested. In fact, I felt proud that, as a physician, I had the right to do something this important, this momentous for this little baby and her parents.

I clicked open the side wall of the incubator and lowered it so that I could reach her more easily than through the twinned circular access hatches. The baby cocooned inside was barely larger than my open hand. As I read the baptismal formula from the book, which the nurse held open for me, I traced the sign of the cross on her minuscule forehead, peeking out from under a crocheted peach-coloured cap. The skin felt moist; it was shiny red and so thin it was translucent. I thought I almost could see her heartbeat. So, this is what being a doctor is, I thought, dealing with matters of life and death. Then I scoffed at myself, embarrassed for being melodramatic, but the feeling of responsibility remained. When I'd finished, after the nurse had bundled the baby – Ava – up again, I laid my hand on the roof of the incubator and found myself saying "Our Father" in my head, the rote Polish of my childhood prayers reassuring.

For the rest of the unusually quiet night, I sat by Ava's incubator, paging through *Smith's Recognizable Patterns of Human Malformation*, a compendium of the most common genetic conditions. Common for genetics, exceedingly rare for pediatrics. This book would become my constant companion over the next three decades – every self-respecting

NICU has a copy. I tried to determine what Ava had, but lacking experience and unable to recognize and name her features, I came up empty-handed. Now, with almost three decades of clinical genetics experience, I am quite sure that Ava had triploidy. Every single cell in her body had an extra set of chromosomes – not an extra single chromosome, like in Down syndrome, but a complete set of twenty-three extra for a total of sixty-nine. Such an excess of genetic material – 50 percent – is incompatible with life. Babies with as little as one extra chromosome 18 or chromosome 13 seldom survive; Down syndrome is an exception and only because it involves the smallest of the human chromosomes.

Although the baby's breaths came less and less frequently as morning arrived unseen in the windowless NICU, her heart was still tracing green waves on the monitor over her head when I stopped at her incubator on my way out the door. I watched her tiny chest lift every thirty seconds or so, but there was no other discernible movement; her face was placid, still. Her eyes were closed – she looked peaceful, wrapped tightly in her blanket, only her tiny red face showing.

When I returned the following day, another premature baby was fighting for its life in the incubator where Ava had lain.

From that night on, *Smith's* became my companion in moments of quiet during my nights on call in the NICU. I would flip through its thick, chalk-overlay pages, stopping at a particularly interesting or disturbing photo with the fascination that I remembered having while at Bloorview. Now, however, I was as much if not more interested in the text accompanying the photographs. A page was dedicated to every condition, several if the disease was better described. Every entry began with a short blurb on the syndrome's discovery, delineation and history; followed by subsections with detailed lists of "Abnormalities," which included an estimate of intelligence level; followed by "Natural History," the occurrence and timing of complications, and death. "Aetiology," the cause of the condition, concluded each entry. In the 1988 edition, the cause was more often than not listed as "unknown."

One night while on call, as I sat at the nurses' station reading the section on otopalatodigital syndrome type 2, a female neonatal fellow peeked over my shoulder and snickered "Guppy!" I chuckled, too – the infant's huge and widely spaced eyes, located almost at the temples, and its tiny puckered mouth hovering over a non-existent chin did make the baby look like a fish viewed head-on. I'm still embarrassed.

As I paged through *Smith's* during rare lulls of NICU on-call nights, two pictures stood out. One was of a boy with a head of thick curls, a tiny jaw and chin, and a rib cage visibly too narrow in circumference, one lone tear hanging off the long lower eyelashes of his right eye. He looked straight into the camera with the reproachful eye of an old, wise soul. His lone tear just broke my heart – he looked as if he hadn't wanted to be examined, probably hadn't wanted to have his photo taken, either, but he only allowed himself that one tear, the look in his eyes a mixture of bravery and sadness. He had cerebrocostomandibular syndrome. The other was a photograph of a naked South Asian–looking boy with underdeveloped genitalia and fused eyelids. Sparse eyelashes poked through the skin on his face where his eyes should have been. He stood with his feet spread wide apart and arms flung out as if to feel where he was standing. It was not his nakedness that bothered me so much, nor the condition itself – Fraser syndrome. It was the setting. The boy stood in an open courtyard of a colonial-looking building in Lucknow, India, scrunching his fused eyelids against the sun's glare that he couldn't see but could probably still feel. I imagined people milling around beyond the frame of the photograph. How shameful. Doubly so – first for it to be taken without, seemingly, any respect for the child, and second for it to be included in four iterations of this venerable textbook. It wasn't until 1997, with the publication of the seventh edition, that the editors finally replaced it with a photograph of a newborn with Fraser syndrome in a hospital incubator.

Many years later, I read Annie Dillard's *For the Time Being*, a book of beautiful, interlinked essays on clouds, sand, Judaic mysticism and, to my surprise and delight, *Smith's Recognizable Patterns of Human Malformation*. When I borrowed Dillard's book from my local library, I had no idea that one of its threads comprised her musings about this textbook. The edition that inspired Dillard was the one I had discovered that night on call in the

NICU – and still refer to, four editions later, at least once a week when diagnosing new patients. Reading Dillard's book, I recognized the patients based on her descriptions alone, so vivid and detailed were they, but what stunned me were the extraneous details that I had never noticed: the white polka-dot collar on the blouse of a girl with frontonasal dysplasia, the hand of a physician or photographer supporting the back of the brother with Seckel syndrome. Incredulous, I pulled out my copy – it sits on my desk next to its four subsequent iterations – to verify her rendition. I shouldn't have doubted her – Dillard was right.

I couldn't believe that I had missed those details when I pride myself on noticing the smallest differences in my patients' appearances. Even as I thought myself so sensitive in my responses to these photographs when I first saw them, I failed to notice the details that made the people in the photographs individuals. Dillard's artistic eye saw those children complete with their clothes and surroundings, while my medical one had honed in on their physical features alone. In the clinic, I comment on the amber beads around a baby's wrist, on their Spider-Man underwear, their stuffies and blankies. But I focus on physical findings – it's my job, after all, which is why it took thirty years and Annie Dillard's exquisite descriptions to make me notice the non-pathologic details in the *Smith's* photos.

Later that week, I bought my own copy of *Smith's* at the University of Toronto Bookstore, knowing that as a pediatrician I would have to know these conditions in detail.

I loved neonatology and its self-contained, quiet world surrounded by the bustle of a large urban adult hospital. Maybe it was the novelty of the residency, maybe it was because I was learning at an amazing rate – not only clinical knowledge and experience but, much more thrilling to master, skills and procedures. I learned to thread a tiny tube into larynxes of babies fifteen weeks premature, and to insert plastic catheters into the veins and arteries in their belly buttons. I learned the physiology of the lungs and their gas exchange much better and faster when I had to monitor the ventilators keeping babies alive than I ever could from lectures. I became an expert at spinal taps in the tiniest babies in the entire city. I didn't even mind the twenty-four-hour shifts on call – at least I could go home the following morning, to crash and sleep until it was time for dinner. During this rotation, Jimm began a lovely ritual that he would follow for the next three years. He always made the bed up before he left for work in the morning so that when I arrived home an hour or so later it waited for me, with crisp, tightened sheets, fluffed-up pillows, the duvet pulled back perfectly on the diagonal – did I mention that in addition to being uncommonly kind, Jimm was somewhat perfectionistic? Often, I would not even change out of my greens but slide between the sheets, blessing whoever invented beds and bed linens and duvets, and fall asleep thinking grateful thoughts toward Jimm.

When I finished that first eight-week rotation in the NICU – with a twenty-four-hour shift on call, no less – Jimm sent me flowers.

☛

At the beginning of residency, every first-year was matched with a third-year – a senior resident – as a mentor. I was so thrilled to be at SickKids, so excited to make new friends that when Cynthia told me she would be mine I blurted out an invitation for dinner.

"No, no," she said quickly, visibly uncomfortable. "It's not like that."

Even the socially inept me recognized that she didn't want to be friends. Soon, I realized that the interns accepted into the program directly from medical school, those admitted to the straight pediatric internship, held a different status as opposed to those of us accepted after a year of a rotating internship. By virtue of not having matched last year, I was already a second-class citizen. On the other hand, a few weeks later, Cynthia, a former straight intern, was chosen as one of two of the next year's chief residents, the highest rank a resident could hold during training.

Cliques formed and, again, I found myself on the outside looking in. The more I wanted to make friends, the more it backfired. I was intelligent enough to realize that it couldn't possibly be a problem with everybody else – the problem, whatever it was, must have lain with me.

Polish immigrants used to say – and probably still do – that we have to be twice as smart to compete with Canadian-borns. Not very original, I know, and I'm sure that all immigrant groups share a version of this sentiment, but my father and his engineer cohorts were convinced of this. Having arrived during the '80s recession, they had witnessed new immigrants being let go after a year or so, often before other employees, their Canadian dream entering a long hiatus while they drove cabs, while dentists worked on a factory assembly line – if they were lucky – and doctors delivered pizzas. Being Polish – with our historically determined doom and gloom, our pessimistic outlook, primed and fostered by the nepotism and cronyism of the Communist Party – we needed an explanation for our perceived failures. I soaked up those sentiments at dinners my parents hosted for their friends, at Christmas parties and at New Year's Eve celebrations, even if deep inside I knew that it really wasn't true. But in medical school, thinking that I didn't get a summer research position or a scholarship because of my foreign name was much more palatable than admitting I wasn't good enough. This conviction bored into me like a worm through a soft, ripe apple.

By the time of my residency at SickKids, I had thought that I'd left those thoughts behind – after all, I did get into the most competitive pediatric residency in Canada. It should have been enough, but when the politics of the residency dawned on me, my old fears and insecurities returned.

☞

After two months of the neonatology rotation confined to the nursery and NICU at Mount Sinai, the rest of my first year at SickKids exploded to cover the basics of general pediatrics: emergency and ambulatory care, general pediatric wards, adolescent medicine clinic, pediatric surgery service – the whole huge academic and clinical world of SickKids. The hospital catered to two distinct patient populations: chronically ill, complex patients with multiple medical and surgical problems who frequently returned and seldom got better; and the general population of the downtown core – well children with acute childhood illnesses. Those were seldom admitted to the wards, and if they were, they were soon discharged. During the day, as a junior resident on the wards, I was responsible for four to six patients. I had to make sure that the orders were carried out by the nurses; that the laboratory results were checked and the abnormal ones reported, discussed and acted on. On nights on call, as juniors we looked after all the patients on our respective wards and admitted those sent up from the emergency department. We had to review all admissions with the senior resident, sometimes as many as ten a night per ward. We didn't get much, if any, sleep on those nights.

Sleep. When I was resident my three most favourite things in the world were sleep, sleep and sleep. As a junior resident, I was seriously handicapped in the sleep department – all my life I had needed an average of at least eight hours of sleep every day. I never pulled all-nighters (except for that one), I seldom studied (or partied) late and if I did, I paid for it over the next day or two. But there is no such thing as eight hours of sleep a night when you are an intern or a resident – at least not when I was a resident. Since then, spurred by the New York City Libby Zion case where an eighteen-year-old woman died as a result of what was believed to be an error by an overworked resident, numerous regulations and legislations have limited the number of hours worked by Canadian residents. Currently, the limit is eighty hours per week – in some rotations during my residency, including the hours on call, we sometimes worked a hundred-plus-hour weeks – and the longest shift allowed is thirty hours.

The pediatric residency tested us with several types of on-call shifts. In the intensive care units, both neonatal and pediatric, we went home after a twenty-four-hour shift whenever the 8:00 a.m. rounds finished. In the emergency department, the longest shift lasted twelve hours overnight, 8:00 p.m. to 8:00 a.m. On those rotations, after handing over my patients in the morning and I would step through the hospital door and suck in the outside air – fresh and crisp after hours spent in the sterile, dry, recirculated atmosphere of the hospital – then walk to the bus, which took me up University Avenue to Eglinton Station, and then walk another three short blocks home along Eglinton Avenue. Once inside our apartment, I would collapse in bed and sleep until Jimm arrived home in the evening. It wasn't until my senior year that I heard that some residents would take those post-call days to run errands and do chores. Such things had never occurred to me – sleep trumped everything.

In contrast, on the wards, we were on call every third or fourth night, which meant coming to work at 8:00 a.m. and leaving by 5:00 p.m. the following day, but more often later. Yes, a thirty-four-hour shift. Sometimes, we managed to nap for an hour or two here and there, most often in a chair, head on the table at the nurses' station, but more often than not we went without sleep for the duration. And since I am unable to sleep unless my trunk is horizontal, I could not catch up during sit-down rounds or teaching sessions, as was the accepted custom (as long as we slept quietly, the joke went), so I never got the benefit of at least a few minutes of REM sleep to recover my cognitive faculties. By the early afternoon of the post-call day, I was liable to say and do stupid things. My prefrontal filter, the requisite social inhibition that barely functioned when I was at my best, fizzled out completely during post-call sleep deprivation. The world became increasingly fuzzy, social niceties less and less relevant, and my eyelids more and more heavy.

It was on a post-call day that I waved a spinal needle at a flailing, scream-ing five-year-old admitted for suspected viral meningitis after I failed to get a spinal fluid sample from him. He thrashed and arched his back after I had inserted the needle between his vertebrae so that the needle bent at almost a right angle, as it weren't stainless steel but plastic. Three nurses were holding him down and this was my third attempt.

"See what you've done?" I hissed at him. It was then that the charge nurse called the senior resident to take over. When she arrived, the senior decided that the spinal tap was not necessary after all, tucked the screaming kid in and let him settle down, all without a word to me.

The next day, our attending took me aside after the morning rounds and asked what had happened. I had no idea that the nurses were upset, that they had reported me, that the senior had corroborated my "unpro-fessional behaviour." Apparently, they had all talked after I'd left the day before and decided to notify the attending, yet nobody said a word to me either day. I was stunned by what I perceived as a betrayal. Why didn't they speak to me first? Why didn't they stop me if my behaviour was so egregious? As it was happening, I could only think that the senior told me to do a lumbar puncture and a lumbar puncture I was going to do. I thought I was doing my job; I wanted to do it right.

"Are you religious?" The attending's question broke through my spiralling thoughts.

"What?" I looked up into her pea-sized eyes, distorted by thick corrective lenses. I thought I misheard her.

"Sometimes religion can help with these matters," she said. "If you have something else to look to other than work." I wasn't sure whether to burst out laughing or burst into tears. She watched my face for a moment and then, as if reaching a decision, walked away, leaving me standing in the hallway.

Thirty years later, I still cringe when I remember what happened that awful afternoon.

In pediatrics, doctors care for patients of three orders of magnitude: five hundred-gram preemies housed in NICU incubators, five-kilogram toddlers crying on the general pediatric wards and sullen fifty-kilogram teenagers in the adolescent medicine clinic. In children, diseases present differently depending on age, so we have to know the variations of disease at every age and stage of human development. Because small bodies have very little reserve for tolerating dehydration or infection, residents have to learn to determine quickly how sick a sick infant is before they become ICU-sick or need resuscitation. Babies and little kids can remain relatively well, their bodies fighting off infection or dehydration for hours, only to become moribund within minutes. It's a question of nuance: an infant with meningitis or a blood infection will not reach out for the truck you dangle in front of his face no matter how colourful and noisy it is. A toddler with appendicitis will not slurp up the Popsicle you offer, even in her favourite flavour. I loved learning those tricks of the pediatrician's trade.

And I loved acquiring knowledge, practical this time; all those years of studying physiology and anatomy were paying off. I started intravenous lines on children of all sizes; I loved hearing the "pop" of the correctly done lumbar puncture. One Friday morning during Chief Rounds – a teaching session led by the chief resident – Paul presented a vomiting six-month-old girl who was brought to the emergency department. On the blackboard, he wrote the results of the baby's blood electrolytes, sampled as she was being resuscitated. Both the calcium and potassium were dangerously low, and the seniors were ready to infuse her with solutions to correct the imbalances – the faster the better; they knew the doses, the composition, the rates of infusion. But both of those treatments were quite dangerous and something didn't feel right to me.

"Wait a moment," I said. Twelve pairs of eyes swung toward me. "These are pretty heavy-duty stuff."

"Yes?" Paul said.

"It doesn't seem right – the kid would be much sicker with these levels. Look, the sodium is lowish, too."

Stony silence. "Where was the blood taken from?" I asked, a light bulb flickering in my head.

Paul allowed himself a smile. "From the vein with the IV," he said.

Bingo! The blood drawn downstream from the IV site was diluted by what was being pumped into the baby's blood. "Draw another sample," I said.

"We did," Paul said. "The 'lytes were normal. You just staved off an iatrogenic cardiac arrest."

From the looks around the room, I had the feeling that some of the seniors were pissed off that a junior had just showed them up. But I didn't care – I was good.

✒

The first year of my residency, Jimm and I managed to fend off my winter blues – as we referred to my funny spells at the time – by going on a week-long holiday in late November to the island of Montserrat: a paradise of black sand beaches and verdant nutmeg and coconut palm trees that crawled up the sides of an active volcano. The landing strip abutted a cliff and stopped a few feet shy of the turquoise-green waves of the Caribbean. The trip worked – no funny spells that winter or spring.

Back at work, during the insanely long days, it was *Star Trek: The Next Generation* on the huge TV screen in the lounge that kept me sane. I had been a Trekker – not a Trekkie! True aficionados of *Star Trek* call ourselves Trekkers; those not in the fold call us Trekkies – ever since Jimm showed me how to watch the original series reruns on the medical school's monitors on Saturday mornings, but it was during the three difficult years of my residency that my obsession peaked. The residents knew that if I was in the lounge, it was *Star Trek* until eight. Of course, I wouldn't insist if hockey playoffs or a baseball game was on – that would be foolhardy. Fortunately, *Star Trek* never interfered with *Seinfeld* or *Friends*. I so wanted to be on the *Enterprise*; I wanted to really, truly belong to an elite group who liked and respected each other. And who liked *me* back.

Some of that came to pass: at the beginning of the year, the first-year residents would get together at the end of every rotation. This tradition did not continue, however, as soon as some cliquey relationships emerged. But another group of us continued to meet, twice or three times a year, well into our fourth year. By and large, we all coped alone: Mike played soccer regularly, Anne painted watercolours, Lynn spent time with friends outside the residency, others were active in their church. I read voraciously to escape the tedium. But all of us felt constantly exhausted, and it might be fair to say that for the first three years of residency our main hobby was sleep.

I did make a friend later that year. Lynn was one of the straight interns but she was not arrogant or competitive – she knew her worth and didn't need to prove it. Throughout the years, she was the one I talked to the most. One year, she and I travelled to St. John's, ostensibly to attend the national pediatrics meeting, but what we really did was rent a car and drive across the Avalon Peninsula to visit Cape Spear and Middle Cove. In town, we hiked the Battery and up Signal Hill. One day, we went on a whale-watching tour, and that evening, I got "screeched in" (Lynn couldn't kiss the cod because of her allergies) and was made an honorary Newfoundlander. What a great conference that was.

☞

In the second year, our rotations took us through the "-ologies." We worked on the subspecialty wards and clinics in cardiology, nephrology (kidney), endocrinology (hormones, but mainly diabetes), respirology (lungs) and immunology where the attending physicians were world leaders in their fields and ran research laboratories. During these rotations, I met patients and their parents, who often knew more about their diseases than I would ever learn. They intimidated me much more than the attendings did. I had studied so long and hard to learn all the pathways, the complications of heart arrhythmias or liver or kidney failure, their treatments and therapy regiments, and here – stretched on a gurney in the emergency room or propped high on pillows in a bed on the ward – an eight-year-old lectured me on his heart's workings better than any cardiac surgeon or cardiologist could. I met mothers who knew the drug interactions of their child's medications backward and forward, and fathers who had replaced fallen out G-tubes more times than I ever would in my lifetime. Woe to the resident who did not pay attention to the mother when she said that her vomiting baby girl should be admitted, or to the father who said his son's wheezing wasn't responding to the inhalers. The patient – and, by extension, their parent – is always right. Ever since, I always tell my patients' parents that they are the experts on their children's diseases in ways that I could never aspire to.

Two months into the second year, I got in trouble again. While on call one night for the endocrinology service, a nurse paged me to the ward to restart an intravenous on a newborn with hypoglycemia – dangerously low blood sugar – whose intravenous cannula had come out. He needed a constant infusion of glucose to prevent brain damage. The good news: I had a window of two, maybe three hours max to restart the intravenous. The bad news: starting an IV on a fat newborn was next to impossible – veins, lost in their fatty padding, rolled away or collapsed when poked with a needle.

That night, after failing three times, I stared at the cute, chubby baby wondering what to do next. Images of him having a seizure from lack of sugar hovered at the edge of my consciousness. Brain damage would be next.

We had no "IV team" in the hospital during nights – none of those amazing nurses with the fingers of angels who could thread an intravenous into a hair if need be.

Then I had the brilliant idea of taking the little guy to the emergency department. Maybe one of the nurses there, much more experienced than I, could get the intravenous in. I told the bedside nurse what I planned, bundled the baby up and headed out of the room past the nurses' station. Nobody spoke to me as I stood in the hallway waiting for the elevator to arrive.

The nurses in the emergency department were not happy with another IV to start. Two tried, but they failed as well. The baby sucked happily on a bottle of glucose solution – I made sure he was getting sugar that way – and was alert in that bright watchful awareness that only a two-week-old can pull off in the middle of the night. After about forty minutes, the emergency room senior finally threaded the intravenous into a vein in his tiny hand and, with a sense of triumph, we connected his line to the glucose solution bag hanging on the pole. During that time, I had answered two or three pages to the other floors I was covering that night. No disasters, just basic scutwork that I was able to handle over the phone. I never left the baby's side.

I bundled him up and – intravenous pole with the swinging plastic bag of glucose solution in hand – triumphantly sauntered back to the floor, the baby's arm securely tucked under his blanket, taped to a padded board, bandaged over and over to prevent accidental dislodgement as the glucose flowed smoothly into his bloodstream.

"I don't want to see this baby ever again," I joked as I handed him back to his nurse. I charted in detail what I had done. It takes only one baby to keep you up all night, I thought as the elevator doors whooshed closed behind me.

At four in the afternoon the next day, as I signed my patients over to the on-call resident, already thinking about my bed, the program director's office paged me. I groaned – what now?

The most terrifying attending, Dr. Robert Ehrlich, the chief of endocrinology, was waiting in the director's office. I did not know at the time that his gruff, prickly exterior hid a heart of gold. He had spent most of his professional career treating children with diabetes. Much later, an endocrinology fellow told me that he treated all his patients as if they were his own kids, that "he only let the parents borrow them for a while," but at the time, all I knew was that he scared the bejesus out of me. The endocrinology charge nurse, a woman my age, sat next to him with what I could only interpret as a smirk on her face. I immediately knew I was in trouble.

The program director told me that the endocrine ward nurses had filed an official complaint about me because I had taken the baby off the ward without following proper procedures. According to the report, I never told anybody where I was going, and the whole time I was off the ward, they had no idea where the baby was and were worried sick about the baby's blood sugars.

"Why didn't they page me?" I asked. "I got several pages when I was in the ER."

"You left the baby unattended?" Ehrlich challenged me.

"There was a phone in the room," I said.

"What if the baby ends up brain damaged because of what you did?" he asked. As if I had not worried about that myself while struggling to start that damn IV.

"I checked his sugar several times in the ER. It was stable," I said.

"The nurses were very worried. One of them cried, she told me," the charge nurse said.

As if. I was sure that the nurses were just happy to nail a female resident. In pediatrics, the resident body was split roughly half and half, and I never gave much thought to there being different standards for male and female residents. I believed in meritocracy and attributed all my trip-ups to my own failings, moral and professional, but my friend Lynn, who was on excellent terms with the nurses, told me how male residents didn't need to clean up after lumbar punctures or after inserting intravenous lines – the nurses did that and other things for the males that the female residents had to do themselves.

"I'm sorry," I said.

All I wanted was to be able to walk the hospital corridor as I had seen a first-year male resident do a few weeks back. He had looked cozy and paternal, yet cool and competent as he carried a baby out the hospital entrance and to Toronto General Hospital across the street – the baby's mother was a patient there and the baby had needed some blood tests done at SickKids. I wanted to appear – no, not appear; *to be* that comfortable and competent, that protective. Instead, here I was being reprimanded by the chief of service, hated by the nurses and with a possibly brain-damaged baby on my conscience.

"I hope you'll never do this again," Ehrlich said.

I was dismissed after being informed that the complaint would be recorded in my file. I never heard anything else about the baby, which I interpreted to mean that he ended up being fine, after all.

➦

After my debacle with the hypoglycemic baby, it became obvious even to an unobservant naïf like me that, at SickKids, more than medical knowledge and skill was required to advance one's career. If I'd had a better relationship with the nurses, indeed if I'd had *any* relationship with the nurses, they probably wouldn't have reported me; they simply would have told me off in private and that would have been that. The associate chief resident on call that night didn't miss a beat distancing herself from me: the following morning she spoke to me and said that had I paged her she would have advised me to drop a feeding tube into the baby's stomach to make sure that he was getting enough glucose while we struggled to insert his intravenous, adding that she had told the program director exactly that when questioned about the incident. "That way you avoid the risk of hypoglycemic brain damage," she finished her lecture.

I never told the other residents about my mishaps with the spinal tap or the hypoglycemic baby. I pretended that nothing had happened and fervently hoped that nobody other than the people involved knew. I'm sure other residents got in trouble the way I did, if only as a chewing out by the ward attending, which happened regularly. Sometimes it was the parents that chewed us out. Once, on morning rounds on the cardiology ward, a mother berated me for what seemed like an eternity: I was a horrible person, I never talked to her, I had been ignoring her son – none of which was true.

Afterward, in the hallway, the female attending said, "Better you than me."

Even if SickKids had the largest rumour mill ever, you never talked about your misdeeds – it was as if by discussing them you admitted that you had deserved the dressing down. But we did talk, and talked a lot, about lawsuits – on average, one resident a year would be named in a lawsuit alleging a medical error. A senior resident who sent a three-month-old girl home from the emergency department, even though the mother requested intravenous fluids; the baby died at home. A junior who did the same thing but to a five-year-old boy; he suffered a cardiac arrest from dehydration at another hospital. Another who inserted a catheter into the artery instead of the vein in a baby's arm; the boy lost a tip of his finger. And I don't know how many residents had complaints lodged with the College of Physicians and Surgeons, but I suspect there were some. We didn't advertise it. In fact, the first piece of advice given to a physician calling the legal protective agency was always not to discuss one's case with anybody.

I was missing the ability to read social cues and had no talent at sucking up, tolerating bullshit or networking. In addition to all that, there was simple luck. Each of these were required in various degrees for success, but I had entered the place thinking that I could conquer it with just my healed brain, hard work and dedication. That's why I tried the lumbar puncture so many times. That's why I carried the baby to the emergency department when I couldn't start the IV myself instead of calling the associate chief resident.

There was also nepotism: a coveted fourth-year associate residency spot went to the son of the incoming new chief of pediatrics. A well-connected second-year resident switched easily between the two most competitive residencies in the city (from pediatrics to radiology and back the following year). There were networks and cliques to which I had no access other than as a witness. And since I still wasn't good at reading Canadian social cues, I often shot my mouth off at the wrong time, which did nothing to advance my cause or win friends.

The spring of that year, I found refuge in the SickKids NICU where I spent eight weeks looking after the sickest babies in the province if not the country. These weren't simply premature babies; they were babies who were premature *and* very sick. By that time, the in-patient wards and the intensive care units had moved to the new Atrium, a nine-storey wing on Elizabeth Street. The NICU, a world unto itself, occupied half of the third floor. I seldom ventured out from its confines, eating lunch in the nurses' lounge there. At nights, the 10:00 p.m. rounds finished, the babies tucked in their incubators for the night – metaphorically speaking, there were no procedures or interventions except for the urgent ones – I wandered the rooms and chatted with the nurses. Sometimes, they would let me feed a baby, one of the bigger and stronger ones, and afterwards I would sit in a rocking chair and have my fill of cuddles.

☛

My second year ended with four awful weeks on the oncology ward. There, a six-year-old girl with an aggressive form of leukemia awaited a bone marrow transplant. Her doctors had identified a donor in the bone marrow registry and were trying stronger and stronger chemotherapy treatments to suppress the cancer in her body so that the transplant could go forward. They never succeeded – the malignant cells killed Olivia before she could get the transplant. In another room, a chubby Ghanaian toddler who made us laugh with his antics wasn't responding to treatment of a supposedly straightforward case of leukemia – we discovered he had AIDS, a death sentence back then. Nicole, a seventeen-year-old First Nations girl, lay dying in constant bone-searing pain from a metastatic neurofibrosarcoma – a massively aggressive cancer of the cells that produce nerve sheaths – that had riddled her brain and spinal cord, and did not respond to ever-increasing doses of morphine. She cried when awake and moaned when asleep. One day, I transferred Aurelio, a boy with Wiskott-Aldrich syndrome, to the pediatric ICU as his mother clung to his stretcher, sobbing. She was the carrier of the condition that predisposed her son to infections and cancer, and she blamed herself for his illness. He never returned to the ward.

That month, I chewed all the cuticles off my fingers – the state of my nail beds is a most reliable indicator of how well or how poorly I am coping with stress. During those four weeks on the eighth-floor oncology ward, I glued Band-Aids on the nail bed of at least one finger almost every day; my throbbing hangnails woke me up at night.

I wrote orders for chemotherapy and morphine, started IVs and stuck needles between vertebrae for spinal taps, all in a haze as I tried to blot out the pain, suffering and death around me. In my own constant state of sadness and upset, I closed off the feeling parts of my brain and pretended to be detached and professional. Inside, my guts twisted with sorrow. I didn't feel that I could confide in anybody and I wasn't aware of any available supports. We had a yearly winter retreat where each year's residents were allowed a weekend off, ostensibly to commune with nature and with each other at an Ontario resort (we picked a different one every year and the hospital paid the expenses). But the retreat was geared more toward corporate team-building and improving performance rather than well-being. While there, we didn't talk about our patients or our mental anguish, and definitely not about personal difficulties. My mantra was "never show weakness, don't give anyone a chance to laugh at you." By then my carapace had hardened into a scaly, tough shell that I pretended repelled off any hurt and disappointment.

➡

In third year, which began July 1, right after the second year ended with some of us on call on June 30, we repeated many of the rotations from the first – wards, emergency, NICU – but this time in the brand-spanking-new SickKids Atrium, the new wing of SickKids that had opened to much fanfare two months earlier. Its wards were spacious and all had large playrooms where doctors were not allowed. All the patient rooms were single with full-length sofa beds for the parents, TV sets and separate bathrooms; many of them opened onto the central space – the eight-storey glass-topped atrium – where a papier-mâché sculpture of an acrobat pig in a lilac tutu balanced over two cows in denim overalls. On the ground floor, colourful murals decked the walls, a harmonium tooted in the corner and olive trees greened in terracotta planters, the latter hastily replaced with ficus after the first Canadian winter killed them off.

The senior year brought much responsibility: we supervised the medical students, interns and first-year residents; we co-signed the medical students' orders; and we were responsible for the care of all the patients on the team. In theory, the attending staff physicians had to be informed about everything, but if and when things went wrong, the final responsibility lay with us. I always felt that I was totally on my own during on-call nights as a senior, that nobody had my back – not the nurses, not my fellow residents, not the associates and definitely not the staff physicians.

In 1991, when I began my training, the atmosphere among the residents was still tainted by a tragedy from ten years earlier when an eight-year-old boy died on the general pediatric ward. Although initially exonerated, in the end both the intern and the senior resident responsible for the boy's care were thrown under the bus by the attending physicians and by the hospital administration after the parents took the case all the way to the Supreme Court of Canada. The residents had only been following the supervising staff physician's and various consultants' recommendations – at least that was what the upper-year residents had told us. The boy had been hospitalized for recurrent vomiting for which a cause wasn't apparent in spite of X-rays, blood tests and specialists' investigations. A psychiatric consultation had been requested by the attending physician and the child psychiatrist had attributed the boy's vomiting to psychological problems. Upon his recommendation, the boy was made to clean up after himself when he vomited. A few days later, shortly after morning rounds, the boy was found to be severely dehydrated. He suffered a cardiac arrest and died in the ICU several days later. His autopsy showed a gangrenous intestine caused by a congenital gut malrotation – a defect where the bowel twists around itself during development. The results of the barium contrast X-ray of his bowels, which had been ordered specifically to detect that condition, had been reported incorrectly by the radiologist.

The parents sued the hospital, the attending physicians, the consultants and all the residents and interns who had anything to do with the boy. The case made news headlines around the country. The year before I began my residency, another round of legal consultants and experts descended upon SickKids to review the case as ordered by the College of Physicians and Surgeons of Ontario. Finally, while I was a second-year resident, the college released its verdict to the public. In the final iteration of its verdict, only the senior pediatric resident and the intern on call that night were held responsible – not the attending pediatrician, not the consultant psychiatrist whose orders they had followed, not the radiologist who had missed the malrotation.

As a result of that verdict, SickKids residents worked with the knowledge that if we made a mistake, the hospital administration and our supervisors would wash their hands of us. We were reminded to pay our dues to the Canadian Medical Protective Association every year because we would have to hire our own lawyers if anything were to happen. Residents were cannon fodder in any potential litigation.

It happened in our year to one of the straight interns. On one of her first shifts in emergency, her first rotation out of medical school, she examined a toddler with gastroenteritis. The child died thirty-six hours later in a peripheral hospital where he had been taken by his parents the following day – he had become so dehydrated that his heart stopped. The resident had reviewed the case with the attending staff physician who had agreed that the child was well enough to go home. After the parents sued the hospital, the resident had to deal with lawyers and court appearances and depositions throughout her entire residency. Her final court appearance would occur five years after having seen the child, when she was a fellow in pediatric cardiology at an American university. She had to fly back to Toronto for it. I could never imagine how she went to work every day with this hanging over her head, and yet she did. She never let on that she was stressed or bothered; she was always pleasant and courteous, smiling and good-natured. I am still in awe of her forbearance and emotional strength – I would have folded seven times every day.

These cases were still in my mind a year later, during my genetics fellowship, when an attending crucified me for "inappropriate" behaviour toward a teenage patient because I had examined his genitalia as part of his annual physical exam during a follow-up visit in the metabolic clinic. The boy's mother supported his claim. Thank god, a pediatric resident was in the room with me – she calmly denied that I did anything wrong or inappropriate and did not back off under the attending's furious glare. In the end, the attending demanded that I write a letter of apology to the boy that, of course, I sent to a Canadian Medical Protective Association lawyer to review first.

One night on call during our senior year, a female resident, a friend, was beaten up by a patient. My friend, all of five-foot-nothing and eighty pounds soaking wet, found herself at the wrong end of a beefy adolescent girl who did not want to be admitted to the ward. Two security guards stood by as the patient pummelled her, blackening her eye, breaking her glasses and cutting her brow, and bruising her ribs. They escorted the patient away, screaming and swearing, only after she backed off by herself – security guards were not allowed to touch a patient. My friend ended up in emergency at Toronto General Hospital across the street for the rest of the night where her injuries were photographed and the cut stitched. The next week, one of the chief pediatric residents asked callously whether my friend would "share her experience" during our weekly teaching rounds. My friend said no.

We were led to believe that this was a price to pay for the privilege of training at the amazing SickKids. Nobody complained, nobody rocked the boat – SickKids could do no wrong. The learning experience – the number of one-of-a-kind cases I saw and treated – equalled none other in the country and fewer than a handful of North American pediatric teaching hospitals. To become a general pediatrician, one could train at many other centres, but for a geneticist-to-be, SickKids was a gold mine of clinical material. Even in the walk-in clinic or the emergency department, I didn't simply look after kids with runny noses; I would listen to the chest of a boy with velocardiofacial syndrome in whom a cold could rapidly become a pneumonia, or palpate the belly of a child with gastroenteritis who also happened to have a complex congenital heart defect that required special modifications to his rehydration protocol. While at times demoralizing, as far as learning went, the residency experience at SickKids was second to none. I would do it all over again in a heartbeat – minus the mistakes, of course.

In August of my third year, I flew to Sioux Lookout for a four weeks' rotation in the Sioux Lookout Zone Hospital, which provided medical care to the Indigenous population of the region.

One day in the white-on-white examining room in the Zone Hospital clinic, I explained to the parents of eleven-year-old Lee that I needed to catheterize her bladder. She'd had several urinary tract infections and had just finished a long course of antibiotics. "We need urine straight from her bladder to make sure that all the bacteria are killed in there," I said. The father left the room after I had finished describing the procedure. I assumed he meant to give his daughter privacy. His wife stayed behind and, as I retrieved the sterile medical tray from the cupboard, stroked her daughter's long, black hair. She said nothing. I told Lee to lie down on the examining table and covered her with a white linen sheet from the waist down. Her hair spread on the pillow, framing her thin face; her brown eyes stared up at me. "It's gonna be okay," I said and patted her leg. "It doesn't hurt." I washed her hairless perineum with a brown iodine solution and spread a blue sterile paper towel over her lower belly. I scrubbed my hands, and just as I was to insert the lubricated catheter into the tiny pink shell of her urethra, the door slammed open and her father barged through.

"Did I tell you that you could do it?" he snapped.

He hadn't. But he hadn't told me that I couldn't, either.

"This is my little girl," he said, pulling up her panties and yanking down her skirt. He scooped her into his arms. "You hurt her. Who do you think you are?"

I thought I was a doctor. But something seemed to have gone wrong and now Lee was not going to get the medically indicated procedure.

The father demanded to see the clinic supervisor.

Neither before nor during my rotation did anybody teach me how to talk and listen to the concerns of First Nations patients. After thirteen years in Canada, I was still grappling with understanding the common Canadian experience, whatever that might be, but I had never failed to communicate medical issues to my patients.

Suddenly, my professional skills were deficient – I knew at that moment that I had missed something vital in my exchange with Lee's father. Both he and I spoke English fluently, yet we had failed to communicate. The medical need for the procedure, its steps and the fact that it wasn't meant to harm the girl had all been lost in translation from the English of a white, Polish immigrant eager to excel at her job to the English of an Ojibwe father who wanted to protect his daughter.

Like many Canadians at the time, I had no idea about the abuse that Indigenous children had suffered at the hands of government doctors and nurses for several generations due to the horrors of residential schools. I had never heard about the Sixties Scoop. As a medical student and resident in downtown Toronto hospitals, I had met homeless and destitute Indigenous patients but knew nothing about the root causes of their disenfranchisement or alcohol and drug abuse. In medical school, an Asian professor had delivered a lecture on Chinese folk medicines, but I only received knowledge of Canadian Indigenous people in passing – we were told they were taciturn and had a high level of tolerance for physical pain, and to account for that during our medical examinations.

Later that day, my supervisor warned me about interpreting the silence of "Indians" as an assent and advised me to always obtain verbal acknowledgement for any procedure. "They don't talk unless you ask a direct question," he said. As I was leaving, contrite and chastised, he told me that the father was having "troubles with the band council" and was looking for a scapegoat. "Take it easy," he offered as his final advice.

Twenty-five years later, all I can say to Lee and her father is: "I am sorry."

➡

I didn't finish my residency with a spotless record with the College of Physicians, either. During an evening shift in the emergency room one snowy February, I examined Tommy, a not-quite-two-year-old boy whose mother was worried that he wasn't well enough to travel to visit his grandparents in Halifax.

"The doctor said he has anemia, but I want to have it checked out," she said. "I'm worried about him."

Tommy did look unwell. He was slurping on his bottle while lying down on the hospital stretcher, sucking in milk in big gulps. Judgment flashed through my mind: baby put to bed with a milk bottle – a sign of poor parenting skills and a risk of tooth decay.

Tommy's skin was pale with that bluish tinge typical of redheads. I examined his skin for bruises, his groin for enlarged lymph nodes – because of the anemia, I was worried that he might have leukemia; he was the right age for it. His gums showed no signs of bleeding. He wasn't dehydrated – I found a thick, wet diaper when I peeled off his blue corduroy overalls. The triage nurse had recorded his blood pressure and pulse as normal, and he had no fever.

"I think he's fine," I said to the mother, but she didn't look convinced.

"I'll check his hemoglobin, if you want," I offered.

She nodded emphatically.

I wrote an order for blood to be drawn for a complete blood cell count and handed it to his nurse. An hour later, after seeing two more patients, I realized that it still hadn't been drawn; the nurse was too busy with other, sicker patients – Tommy had been triaged as "stable" – so I decided to draw the blood myself. Residents didn't usually draw blood in the emergency department – nurses took care of the tests, allowing us to keep seeing patients – but Tommy had waited too long already. His mother would appreciate my gesture.

When his blood tests came back with a normal hemoglobin level – no anemia – and with a normal white count – no evidence of leukemia – I reassured the mother that he was well enough to travel and discharged him from the emergency department. I also told her to come back if she was still worried.

Three weeks later, Dr. Anna Jarvis, the chief of the emergency department, called me into her office.

"Do you remember the boy with diabetic ketoacidosis?" she asked.

"What boy with diabetic ketoacidosis?"

"That's right. You missed it," she said. "He presented at a Dartmouth hospital in a diabetic coma. You're lucky they resuscitated him in Halifax. I just got off the phone with his mother. She said that if she had a gun and met you in the hallway, she'd shoot you."

I gaped at her, dumbstruck. Missed diabetic coma, a death threat – I wasn't sure which was worse. The chief sat behind her massive oak desk, calm and composed in her starched white coat.

"The mother said that you've robbed her of her confidence as a mother and that she will never forgive you," she continued. "That she believed your assurances even though she knew that there was something wrong with her son. I'm telling you this to warn you. Where I come from, we take such threats seriously." She had trained in Kingston, Jamaica.

And that was all she said to me.

I was terrified. Not only had I missed an important diagnosis – thank god the boy was alive and well – but now my life was in danger? What was I supposed to do? Never again set foot at the hospital? Transfer to another program in another city? If I saw the mother down a hallway, should I run away?

A few weeks later, I pulled the dreaded notice from the College of Physicians and Surgeons of Ontario from my mailbox. I had to write a statement, which, of course, I prepared with the help of a lawyer. In the end, based on my notes and an expert opinion, the College determined that I was not at fault – as an inexperienced resident, I could not be faulted for missing the very early stage of diabetes in a toddler. Worst was the knowledge that had I checked his urine for sugar or added glucose level measurement to his blood work, I would have diagnosed his diabetes.

But there had been no reason to do that – the chief complaint had been anemia, and no other red flags appeared on the history or during the physical examination. And even if I had done so, it wouldn't have been a big deal – nobody would have known what could have happened because nothing *would* have happened. I wouldn't have been a hero; I would have been only doing my job. Such a minuscule decision, such enormous consequences. The hospital rumour mill churned: I heard that one of the endocrinologists claimed that I should've noticed that the boy's diaper was soaked, to which Dr. Jarvis had countered that it had been gastroenteritis season and everybody was happy if a child had a wet diaper – it meant that he wasn't dehydrated. There had been no reason to dip his urine for sugar.

I never saw Tommy or his mother again, although two years later I noticed his name hanging on the door to a patient's room on the endocrinology ward – he must have been admitted for a decompensation of his diabetes. I avoided her, although now I think that I should've met with and talked to her, allowed her to rage at me – after all, she had almost lost her son because of my oversight. I would have liked to have had the chance to say that I was sorry. But I was terrified – of her righteous anger, of her grief and, coward that I was, of rocking the boat.

Throughout my residency, I never admitted weakness, never asked for help. Not with medical knowledge or clinical skills, of course, I asked for help with those; I wasn't arrogant. I learned by asking questions. But emotionally I didn't let anybody too close.

So, I struggled with my temper and moods with only Jimm's help. Most days, I managed to remain calm and professional, but that was due to an enormous internal struggle nobody knew about. People noticed the fraction of the time when I snapped at nurses, when I stomped off from rounds to arrange a gastroscopy that a junior resident failed to secure, when I cracked a joke nobody understood or found funny; they did not know how hard I was trying every day, every hour, every minute to stay calm and collected and polite and professional. It was as if constricting hoops, like those on a wooden wine barrel, held me together and pinched my soul every second of the day. I held my breath; I chewed off my cuticles. My neck and shoulder muscles were taut and sore. I wonder what my blood pressure was. I tried so hard and yet most of the time I felt I failed to live up to the standards of an affable resident.

I never wanted to be an associate resident – the fourth-year general pediatric resident. I did apply for it, as was the custom, but apart from the fact that I knew I wouldn't get the prestigious position, I also thought it would be a waste of time given my chosen career. I didn't want to be a general pediatrician who dealt with colds and diarrhea and vomiting and routine well-baby checkups day in and day out. Those had been interesting in Dr. Driver's office, but the novelty wore off rapidly during my ambulatory pediatric rotations in the first year.

And that was why in July, after my second year, I applied for the genetics fellowship at SickKids. I think that the interview with Joe Clarke and Dr. Teresa Costa, the program director of the newly established medical genetics residency, might have been a formality – I had been an almost constant fixture in the genetics department since medical school and nobody else in my year applied for the position. And while this acceptance was not as huge a high as getting that phone call from Alan Goldbloom three years earlier, I was thrilled and excited to be getting ready to study those weird and wonderful diseases, to hunt those zebra diagnoses nobody else knew about, and to do it at the hospital that practically invented clinical genetics in Canada.

It wasn't a constant struggle for those three long years. There were rotations where I soaked up knowledge and gained skills as if without effort, and nights when I got three hours of uninterrupted sleep – a luxury! There were adorable toddlers and grateful parents, many more spinal taps and intravenous starts that went well, and many days when my skills and knowledge were recognized. Once, as a senior pediatric resident, I had to finger-extract stone-hard feces from the rectum of a constipated five-year-old boy. He screamed and the stool clanged as it hit the metal bedpan, but later that day he gave me a toothy smile when I saw him in the playroom, his pain all but forgotten. The most satisfying procedure I ever performed was the reduction of a "pulled elbow," an injury that happens when a caregiver yanks a small child up by the arm. One of the forearm bones dislodges from the elbow joint capsule and the child screams and completely refuses to use that arm. The treatment is ridiculously easy: cradling the elbow in question in one palm you straighten the arm, stretching it, and then force it flexed, all in one smooth motion. The child bawls bloody murder as you do it, and the parent wants to slug you, but the moment you show the boy or girl a freezie, they reach to grab it with the formerly immobile arm and a smile blossoms on their face when they realize it doesn't hurt anymore. As a senior in the emergency department, I tried to put my name next to as many pulled elbows as I could, especially when I needed cheering up.

➤

One February during my third year, my father-in-law didn't go to work, which was enough for Jimm and me to know that he was very ill. At eighty-six, he still rode the subway to his office at Bloor and Spadina and in forty years had never missed a day of work on account of illness. He was diagnosed with chronic myelogenous leukemia and died in early April. His illness coincided with another depressive episode that March, but I was on an easy, no-call rotation in rehabilitation medicine at Hugh MacMillan Centre, which was quite bearable. With my father-in-law's illness I thought I had a reason to be depressed and I muddled my way through the slow days. I only asked for two days off for his funeral.

➤

Toward the end of the year, the third-years began forming study groups to prepare for the final fellowship exam held the following June. I was terrified that I would be left to fend for myself, but I was lucky enough to be welcomed into a group with five amazing and helpful humans who happened to be residents in my year: Lynn, Mannie, Raymond, Abya and Anne. Those five people cared enough about me to tell me off and set me straight. I loved studying with them. I cared whether they passed, too, and wanted to help them. In July, Lynn, Mannie and Raymond became associates (but not the arrogant, don't-you-know-who-I-am? type that I detested so much), and they were able to teach us the minutiae of general pediatrics that the rest of us might have missed or forgotten. Later that year, when I became a fellow in genetics, I grilled them on the principles of inheritance and the treatment of metabolic diseases; Anne did the same with infections – she began an infectious disease fellowship; and Abya with medications, drug interactions and their side effects, as he was a clinical pharmacology fellow. We met twice a week in the evenings when our combined call schedules allowed. Those were the best times of my residency.

We wrote the Canadian fellowship exam in Varsity Arena during two rainy days in September, and on the Saturday morning of the Canadian Thanksgiving weekend, Mannie drove us in a rented minivan to Chicago to write the American Academy of Pediatrics exam, Lynn sleeping in the back seat because she had just finished a twelve-hour associate call. We were so well prepared that instead of reviewing the day before, we toured the Art Institute of Chicago and the Shedd Aquarium, and rode up the Sears Tower. We also cruised the Chicago River in a sightseeing barge, Raymond filming the whole trip.

When we all received the letters saying that we had passed the written Canadian exams and the American board certification, the time came to prepare for the dreaded Royal College fellowship oral exam. Thirty percent of those who took this exam failed.

My study group taught me not to lapse into profanity when I got upset – at the time, I was going through a phase of trying to shock people with choice cursing – because I might forget myself during the actual exam. Abya was coached not to say "pee" and "poo" when answering exam questions. Raymond needed a dose of confidence to speak up, and Mannie to slow down his torrent of words and to stop addressing the parent as "Mom." We psyched each other out and asked nastily difficult questions, all to inure ourselves to the pressure cooker of the actual oral.

To spur ourselves on even more, we repeated horror stories that circulated from previous years: a resident fainting when asked, on her way out, to identify a vein in a patient's neck; an examiner failing a candidate for not washing his hands. Sitting around a battered faux pine table in a conference room at the back of the general pediatrics ward, we kept each other going when we flagged. The actual oral exam consisted of: a long case where one examiner watched you gather the medical history and examine a patient, followed by a presentation to a second examiner who didn't know the patient, and then questions from both of them; a short case, usually a child with a complex medical history whom we had to examine for specific findings; and four shoebox questions, so-called because of the cardboard box in which the chief examiner carried the five-by-seven index cards with the examination topics.

We grilled each other on the last two, but to prepare for the long case, the tradition at SickKids was to ask attendings to practise cases with us, taking the medical history and examining the patient while under their watchful eye and then discussing the case with them. "Get the person who scares you the most because you will never be as anxious as during that final oral" was the advice we'd heard from previous successful candidates. That would have to be Ehrlich, I thought immediately. I was still so scared of him that I didn't even look him in the eye when I asked him to supervise a practice oral with me. To my dismay, he agreed.

"You'll do fine," he said after I finished. And he smiled as if he had recognized my paralyzing terror. All I could do was nod and thank him. That day, I realized that if I could do a long case with Bob Ehrlich watching my every move, I could pass the pediatric fellowship oral.

Come the following June, all six of us passed the orals and became Fellows of the Royal College of Physicians of Canada. As it turned out, we were the only study group at SickKids to accomplish that feat that year.

6.

"No woman in her right mind wants to see a geneticist when she's pregnant," Dr. David Chitayat said when I arrived in his office on the first day of my genetics fellowship. I smiled uncertainly at this gallows humour: beneath the surface jocularity hid a boulder of truth.

For two years starting Monday, July 2, 1994, I split my time between SickKids, where I saw patients in the outpatient genetics clinic and provided consultations in clinical and metabolic genetics on the hospital wards, and Mount Sinai Hospital and Toronto General Hospital, where I was a fly on the wall in the prenatal diagnosis clinic. Apart from the clinical rotations, I also rotated through diagnostic laboratories where I was to learn the basics of molecular tests for specific genetic conditions; of cytogenetics, the study of chromosomes and their anomalies; and of biochemical tests for metabolic diseases – my favourite lab of all.

David Chitayat was in charge of the prenatal genetics service at Toronto General and Mount Sinai. I had met him during my residency genetics rotation, but I remembered only a whirl, a vortex of energy, like the cartoon Tasmanian Devil. As residents, we joked that he ran on a totally different set of batteries; as a fellow, I was awed by his stamina and energy, not to mention his encyclopedic knowledge. He answered emails at 3:00 a.m.; from 8:00 a.m. to 6:00 p.m. he attended to patients in three hospitals – the General, Mount Sinai and SickKids – and was frequently sighted dashing either along or across University Avenue; and he published twenty papers a year – there had never been a genetics conference at which he and his team did not present several papers. His memory for genetics conditions was beyond legendary – it was as if he had stashed, somewhere in his cortex, the entire photo collections of the London Dysmorphology Database and POSSUM (Pictures of Syndromes, Signs and Unknown Malformations), the searchable databases of photographs of genetic conditions we used every day to diagnose patients.

At the many unknown diagnosis sessions that I had attended over the years, he was the most likely to identify a syndrome that nobody else had thought of, and his diagnosis would almost always turn out to be correct. He analyzed patients' photos at the speed of light. Once, I watched him think as he reviewed photographs of my patient, an overweight ten-year-old boy with extra toes and impaired vision; he scanned the photos and, in a matter of seconds, pronounced it "Bardet-Biedl syndrome." It had taken me forty minutes of searching for and cross-referencing the boy's features in several textbooks and atlases to come to the same conclusion, but I was ecstatic that he agreed with my diagnosis. As if all that wasn't enough, he had the gentlest and kindest way with patients and parents. He never gave up on the search for the correct diagnosis, and if he could not find one, he would publish the case in the hopes that other geneticists and patients might benefit from his observations. Of course, he had a syndrome named after him – two, actually. He was too brilliant to think of emulating, but I decided to try anyway.

◗

One of the patients that first day was a pregnant woman referred by her family doctor because her cousin had died from cystic fibrosis. The woman had only recently realized that she was pregnant and was fifteen weeks along; we didn't have much time to determine if she carried the cystic fibrosis gene or to test her baby if she did. At that time, terminations of pregnancy were easily available only up to a certain point in the pregnancy – determining the risks and establishing a diagnosis in prenatal genetics was frequently a race against time.

She was my age. She had a shaggy haircut and was wearing too-tight blue jeans. She had a strong Québécois accent and David had to repeat many phrases to her, but I still don't think she understood him very well. She showed no interest in any type of prenatal testing, nor did she want to know whether she was a carrier for cystic fibrosis, not even when David explained that she had a one in four chance of being a carrier. No, her husband didn't want the test either, she said.

Then David asked her where in Quebec she was from.

"Lac-Saint-Jean–Saguenay," she said.

David glanced at me. I knew what that meant – she had a very high risk of being a carrier for a number of severe genetic conditions endemic to the Charlevoix-Saguenay region: Tay-Sachs disease, a lethal neurodegenerative disease that killed children before their third birthday; tyrosinemia type 1, a defect in the metabolism of the amino acid tyrosine that caused liver failure; and a type of degenerative ataxia. The Francophones who had settled on the shores of the placid Lac-Saint-Jean in the 1830s originated from Charlevoix, which in turn had been populated by the descendants of some six hundred French settlers from Perche in Normandy, among them carriers for these conditions. As their descendants married almost exclusively their French-speaking neighbours, those mutated genes had wormed their way through generations and increased in frequency.

David explained all that to our patient, but she shrugged, an uncertain smile on her face. She did not want tests for diseases she had never seen or heard of.

Why did David tell her about all those diseases? I wondered. She was referred for cystic fibrosis and yet he'd dumped on her the entire genetic burden of her population. Why would he scare her like that? I watched the young woman's face and her baffled eyes, and felt she, too, was wondering: "What do these diseases have to do with me?" It was my first experience of genetic counselling – a crash course – and I thought at first that telling the patient about all those diseases was too much, too scary and irrelevant. But I soon learned that geneticists evaluated their patients for chances of genetic conditions based on their family history, on their ethnic and geographical origins, and on their own reproductive history. They did not solely concentrate on what the consultation requested. The patient needed to know how all those factors could affect her baby, and know the risks that she and her partner faced before she made any decisions about her pregnancy. She had the right to know, especially if a prenatal test was available. What if the baby later did develop one of those horrible diseases and we had not advised her about the risks? But lacking experience, that day, I thought David's actions were cruel and unnecessary.

The central tenet of genetic counselling is "non-directive counselling." The physician or counsellor are obliged to provide the patient with all the available information and all the known risks, no matter how low those risks are, but not to offer advice on what to do. The information has to be presented neutrally, in a detached and measured way, without a trace of guidance or influence. Only the patient has the right to decide whether to test herself, whether to test her baby and – if the results showed that the fetus was affected – to decide whether to stop or continue the pregnancy. Geneticists are trained to not give weight to any of the options, to avoid telling the patient what to do.

"Whatever your decision is, we will support it" is the geneticists' and genetic counsellors' mantra.

At that time, prenatal diagnosis was still a relatively new field. First uses of ultrasound to demonstrate anomalies in a fetus date to the 1950s, but it wasn't until the 1970s that real-time sonograms became more widely employed for this purpose. Amniocentesis was first described in 1955 as a means of obtaining fetal cells for the diagnosis of chromosomal imbalances. Amniocentesis also allowed for the diagnosis of other genetic conditions because the fetal cells could be used as a source of fetal DNA for testing. The two types of prenatal testing are prenatal screening and prenatal diagnosis for a known genetic condition. Prenatal screening identifies the risk of a chromosomal imbalance such as Down syndrome or trisomy 18, and of neural tube defects based on biochemical markers in the mother's blood during the first trimester of pregnancy; when the risk is deemed high enough, diagnostic testing follows. This type of screening was introduced in the late 1980s and was in wide use by the time I began my training. Prenatal diagnosis, on the other hand, determines with certainty – diagnoses – a condition that has previously occurred in the family.

The main consequence of prenatal diagnosis is to allow the pregnant woman the option to end any pregnancy where a genetic disorder or major fetal anomaly is present – a unique and, for many, problematic solution with moral implications for abortion and disability rights.

One day, trying to keep up with David on rounds (he ran on only one speed: super-charged), I followed him as he rushed through a metal door painted a bright yellow. I found myself unexpectedly in a large, windowless room, its formaldehyde smell bringing back memories of first-year anatomy dissections. In the middle of the floor stood a stainless steel table with raised edges, its top sloping toward a drain, its shiny surface reflecting the buzzing fluorescent lights above. An articulated tap was suspended over it like the arm of a skeleton. The walls of the room bulged with plastic containers, bulbous purple-grey shadows floating murkily inside. I was in the autopsy suite.

The full-height, stainless steel refrigerator hissed as David pulled it open. He lifted a small bundle wrapped in a green surgical towel from a shelf in the middle. As he unwrapped it, I saw a fetus no longer than his palm, its tiny hands folded over its chest, a hospital bracelet hanging off its left foot. Its red translucent skin glistened, the lights reflected on its hairless skull. I knew that if I touched it, it would be sticky. Its eyes were still fused. I stood there, frozen, my heart banging in my chest, but I did not gasp, did not blink – it would not have been professional. David briefly examined the baby's mouth, anus, genitalia (female), hands and feet. "Trisomy 18, nineteen weeks," he said as he gently and carefully rewrapped the fetus and returned it to the fridge. I let out the breath I didn't know I had been holding.

After two weeks on the prenatal genetics service, I decided that I did not like it. Not because of the non-directive counselling rule or the life-and-death-before-life-starts dilemmas – as a fellow still in training, I was insulated from the decision-making angst and turmoil – but because in the prenatal clinic, the patients were pregnant women and their partners. All adults. It was disorienting after three years of only having infants, children or teenagers as my patients. And since I had already decided that I would concentrate on metabolics, those biochemical disorders that had always fascinated me and affected mainly children, I knew that there would be very little prenatal genetics. But whoever arranges our path in life laughs at our wishes.

During the genetics fellowship, our teachers drilled into us the need to make the correct diagnosis. "Diagnosis" has two meanings. One refers to the process of seeking clinical clues – the symptoms from history and the signs from examining the patient, weighing the evidence, forming a hypothesis as to what we might be dealing with, and finally formulating the differential diagnosis and eliminating diseases by ordering and interpreting diagnostic tests. The required thoroughness is inherent in the word itself: *dia* – through or thorough – and *gignŏskein* – to learn to know. But the product of such an investigation is also called "diagnosis" – the name of the disease, the condition, the syndrome. Diagnosis implies that the physician making it, after going through the process of diagnosis, discovered something important about the patient and named the complex constellation of findings and features. At a deeper level, establishing a correct diagnosis provides the framework for all subsequent medical interactions and decisions.

There is something metaphysical about naming a condition.

"We need a consult on a newborn with a heart defect and Hirschsprung's disease," I heard once while on the phone with a neonatologist. "The prenatal ultrasound showed agenesis of the corpus callosum."

"Mowat-Wilson syndrome," I blurted out, and the neonatologist inhaled quietly. The unknown had been conquered by naming it. Now we knew what to do, what to expect. Even if my initial impression was wrong, at least the diagnostic workup could proceed. The unknown was scary, especially in a newborn and especially when the baby appeared clearly abnormal.

But to be useful, a diagnosis must be both accurate and specific. For example, the label "multiple congenital anomalies" is devoid of useful information – there are myriad combinations of hundreds of birth defects that could fit this description. Add to that various degrees of intellectual disability and neurologic impairment, and you will see how useless it is: it provides no information about the etiology or the prognosis, the future course of the disease. But when that worthless epithet is replaced with the diagnosis of, say, Costello syndrome, the doctors know what other birth defects to look for and whether to expect developmental delays or medical complications. Once we know the underlying cause – a mutation in the HRAS gene in the case of Costello syndrome – we can also correctly determine the chance of recurrence in the child's siblings or in their own children, and offer a prenatal diagnosis if the parents wish it during their next pregnancy. Making the diagnosis constitutes the most important step in providing care and counselling. That's why geneticists obsess about making not *a* diagnosis, but the *right* diagnosis. A wrong diagnosis is worse than no diagnosis because it leads to false assurances, wrong treatment and potentially the birth of other affected children.

Woe to the geneticist who does not recognize a diagnosable disease. How many times have I heard "The parents were denied the option" of deciding whether to have another child with a diagnosable condition. If the correct diagnosis isn't made in a timely fashion, there is always the possibility of recurrence in the family. Without a correct diagnosis, prenatal diagnosis would be impossible and parents would not have the option of stopping such pregnancies from continuing to term, if they so wish. If, diagnosis made, the parents decide to continue a pregnancy, that is their choice, but they have the right to know what they are dealing with. And as a geneticist, I have the obligation to provide all the information to them to make a fully informed choice. No ifs or buts about it. The need to make the correct diagnosis shapes the way geneticists practice – sometimes we do not stop investigating patients for years.

So, I concentrated on diagnoses and the overarching goal: to prevent the birth of more affected children in families who already have or have had a child with a genetic condition. The search for the right diagnosis drives all the investigations, photo-taking, the diagnostic unknowns sessions at conferences. Geneticists not only chase zebras – those elusive, one-of-a-kind diagnoses – we make sure that their stripes match the exact pattern we need.

Correct diagnosis also allows geneticists to predict the severity of a disease and to tell the parents, in broad strokes, what to expect. At least, in theory. Once, during my residency, when I was still a junior on a general pediatric ward, I stood by the bedside of a two-month-old baby girl just diagnosed with Wolf-Hirschhorn syndrome and listened in horror as one of the more dysfunctional staff geneticists counselled the parents. At two months of age, the baby weighed only four pounds and did not track with her eyes, did not focus on faces; her tiny head flopped on the stalk of her neck when her mother lifted her. Even the medical students in attendance could recognize the severity of her delays. High-arched eyebrows met over a prominent ridge of bone that extended between her eyes onto the bridge of the nose, producing the "Greek-helmet appearance" characteristic of the condition. The baby had been hospitalized to evaluate her feeding problems and poor weight gain, or, in medical lingo, why she was "failing to thrive."

"She will be herself" and "she will show you how far she'll go," the geneticist burbled as she danced around the obvious.

After about ten minutes of these verbal gymnastics, the father lost his patience.

"Will she graduate high school?" he snapped.

"Everybody graduates high school these days," the attending trilled, beaming beatifically. I suppressed an overwhelming urge to kick her in the shin. The father, too, looked like he wanted to slug her. I knew – and I knew the attending knew – that this girl would never learn to talk, would never walk on her own; that she would forever have the abilities of a one-month-old. The developmental trajectory of children with Wolf-Hirschhorn syndrome was well-delineated. He wanted an honest answer and the geneticist never gave it.

Right there and then I promised myself never to prevaricate when it came to the diagnosis or prognosis of a genetic syndrome.

During the second year of my fellowship, I devoted most of my clinical time to metabolic genetics. The clinical application of biochemistry was what I had wanted to do since discovering the subspecialty in my genetics course in medical school. Metabolics, as it was called, was, at the time, the only subspecialty of genetics where physicians could actually do something to alleviate disease. Metabolic genetic diseases are caused by deficiencies of crucial enzymes in the body that cause blocks in the biochemical pathways. Just like an accident on the 401 results in a pileup behind it, these enzymatic blocks lead to a buildup of toxic metabolites which in turn harm important organs such as the liver or the brain.

In other enzyme blocks, just like the trucks that cannot deliver their goods past the highway pileup, certain key molecules are not delivered to tissues that require them and the resulting deficiencies also cause disease. Medications and special diets are geared to prevent these chemical imbalances and, in many cases, prevent brain damage and intellectual disability. Phenylketonuria is one such disease, a success story of metabolic disease therapy. It is the most common biochemical cause of intellectual disability, and, if diagnosed in the first week of life, its effects can be prevented by starting a restricted diet. In order to ensure early diagnosis, newborn screening for phenylketonuria was introduced in the 1960s and has prevented intellectual disability in countless patients.

Metabolics is an intensive and time-consuming specialty – one sick patient with a metabolic disorder can keep a team of physicians, nurses, dieticians and laboratory technicians busy for days on end – but is very rewarding, like when a boy with maple syrup urine disease who was delirious and vomiting uncontrollably two days earlier left the hospital smiling and waving at the nurses. Or when the elevated ammonia in the blood of a girl with a urea cycle disorder normalized and she woke up from her coma, her faculties unscathed. But there are also many diseases that are incurable and relentlessly progressive, and that have robbed children of their abilities and health, and, ultimately, their lives.

A little girl with the most beautiful olive skin and a head full of long, silky black curls was admitted to the diagnostic investigation unit. Her pediatrician referred her for a genetics assessment because of a developmental delay – at eight months old, she did not roll, she did not sit, her head still wobbled. On the genetics investigation unit, she endured needle pokes, a brain MRI and a skin biopsy without so much as a whimper.

As I examined her, I noticed a strange curve to her thin wrist. One of the bones in the forearm – the ulna – flared out in a scooped-outward sway, too large to cradle the bones of her wrist. I've seen this somewhere, I thought.

But in the genetics fellows' room, *Smith's* had nothing to say about it. Of course, whatever condition the girl had would not be represented there; she was not dysmorphic. On the contrary, her face was beautiful, proportionate, symmetrical. But I knew I had seen that wrist somewhere.

Then I remembered: *Nelson Textbook of Pediatrics*, the book I had done my best to memorize during my pediatric residency. On the bottom of page 350, in the section on lysosomal storage disorders, I found a photo that could have been of the girl's wrist. The disease was called Farber's lipogranulomatosis, only forty cases reported worldwide – quite the zebra. Convinced that she had it, I read the description of how it presented and what complications it caused, and went back to examine her again for the skin nodules the textbook said were diagnostic. But she had none on her soft pink skin.

My supervisor on the metabolic service scoffed when I told her about Farber's – it was too rare to be believed – so I lugged the textbook to her office.

"Her wrist looks exactly like this," I said, pointing to the photograph.

The supervisor shrugged her shoulders dismissively.

When the ophthalmologist dilated the girl's pupils, he found the worst possible sign an eye examination can find: a cherry-red spot at the back of each eye, a diagnostic sign of a neuronal storage disorder. Tay-Sachs, Sandhoff and Niemann-Pick diseases all have cherry-red spots and all are horrific neurodegenerative conditions that cause deafness, blindness, paralysis and childhood death. The spot forms when the nerve cells of the retina swell up with undigested lipids. The normally pearly retinal cells become opaque and thick, and obscure the blood vessels at the back of the eye, which normally give the retina its lovely cerise hue and the red eye of flash photography. In the area of the cherry-red spot, the normal blood vessels shine through but the dull grey neurons surrounding its brightness impart an angry, sick look. The sickness is the pale greyness of the entire retina, not the cherry-red spot, but the spot is what scares us when we find it.

"Can't jump to conclusions," my supervisor said, even though she did finally admit that the wrists did resemble the photo in the textbook. "We have to rule out the more common causes of cherry-red spot."

She was right. Only a single lab in North America studied Farber's disease and we had a diagnostic lab for all the other lysosomal diseases right at SickKids. But my gut told me that I was right.

A few months later, at the annual American Society of Human Genetics conference in Montreal, I had dinner with the director of the lysosomal storage disorders lab at SickKids. I mentioned the little girl during dinner in an auberge in Old Montreal. By then, a research lab in Wisconsin had confirmed the diagnosis that I had proposed.

"Great case," John said. "Much credit to your supervisor."

My mouth hung open. "What?"

"Kudos to her for persistence. The first case at SickKids."

"I made that diagnosis," I said.

The director looked puzzled. "She never said," he said and took a sip of his wine.

❧

During the second year of my fellowship, a five-year-old girl with another lysosomal storage disease entered the final stage of her disease. Her bone marrow, choked by lipid-laden cells, finally failed. Her liver and spleen grew huge in her little belly in an attempt to produce the blood cells her bone marrow couldn't. She lay there, her tummy bloated, her arms and legs wasted twigs. She did not cry; she did not complain. One of the mercies of storage diseases that affect the brain is that pain perception fails just like all its other functions. During the course of her illness, she had developed several complications not previously reported in the medical literature. My supervisor allowed me to be the first author of the case report. But, as required by the journal's editorial policies, before we could publish the case, the girl's parents had to agree and to sign a consent form to that effect. Like many parents of severely sick and dying children, they wanted to help others, to put information about the rare disease out there, so they agreed immediately. But I worried that we were exploiting their desire for something good to come out of their daughter's illness.

I felt like shit.

"It is very important to share," my supervisor told the parents. "It may help other families."

The mother wiped her eyes. "Her life won't be in vain?" she asked.

I knew that it was unlikely that the publication of a single case would help another patient. We were only publishing the case because it would look good on our academic records, and would help secure an academic promotion for the supervisor and an academic position for me. I had already absorbed the academic creed of "publish or perish." My supervisor and I were simply getting our names on a peer-reviewed article that might infinitesimally increase genetic knowledge but would not lead to any groundbreaking discoveries. Everybody did it. Everybody, that is, who wanted an academic career.

I thanked the parents as they signed their names on the publication consent form.

I felt like a fraud, but at home that night, I booted up my desktop and wrote the draft of the case report. I was advancing my academic career on the back of a child's illness, on her family's suffering, on that awful genetic toss of the coin. As I wrote the girl's medical history, her personality and beauty – her all-too brief life – ended up buried under a heap of medicalese: genetic tests, brain scans, skin biopsies and X-rays.

It was the first of many such articles I would write and publish. As expected of a clinical genetics fellow who wanted an academic career, I authored several others during my fellowship. I was getting ahead, academically speaking, while the parents suffered through sleepless nights, the beeps of heart monitors and piles of medications to administer. While they made arrangements for their daughter's funeral, I spell-checked my manuscript and labelled photos of their dead daughter's tissues before mailing them to the publisher. I did it for the sake of my academic advancement and the advancement of genetic knowledge, no matter how minuscule it might have been but I can't say that I felt great about it.

☛

Since the summer research project after third-year medical school with Joe Clarke, I had emulated him as best I could. I even bought a Lamy fountain pen and taught myself English cursive; by the time I started my fellowship, my handwriting had become regular and even. And because I wanted to become an academic geneticist who taught medical students, residents and fellows, I knew that I would need a teaching slide collection. With his permission, I and the three other genetics fellows ordered copies of the photographs of the patients we saw in clinics or on the wards.

"Do you have slides of Duchenne's?" we'd ask each other, reverting to disease-specific shorthand in the privacy of the fellows' room. "What about a cherry-red spot? I got a great one yesterday." "That hair-cartilage dysplasia was really interesting; we got all the X-rays on slides." "I have a great photo of the fingertip pads in Kabuki syndrome, saw a patient last week, it was soooo cool" – that last statement from me. I loved it when a single finding would identify a disease – the pathognomonic sign, that telltale clinical finding that cinched the diagnosis.

For my teaching slide collection, I ferreted out photographs illustrating such findings for as many syndromes as I could, as well as microscopy slides of distorted cells and tissues, X-rays of bone disorders, and CT scans and MRIs of the brain. I imagined myself teaching medical students and residents, sharing the excitement of finding the right diagnosis. And even though a voice sometimes niggled at the back of my mind, questioning the ethics of what I was doing, I continued to amass my teaching slide collection, making it as complete, as definitive as possible.

I had become a collector of diseases.

☛

Jimm and I had agreed not to have children during residency. It was too busy a time for both of us; we were dedicated to our training and wanted to do a good job. Add to that my funny spells and my difficulties with temper, and we knew that I would not be able to handle a baby and all the attendant demands of motherhood on top of a residency. I was amazed by the few women who did have children during residency – I had no idea how they managed to do it all. But by the time I passed my pediatric fellowship exam in 1994, I began to think about having a baby. I thought about it a lot. I was ready.

I had always planned to check my carrier status for two conditions before getting pregnant: thalassemia – a form of genetic anemia common in the Mediterranean basin, because of Jimm's Greek ancestry; and Tay-Sachs disease – not because either of us was Jewish but because I wanted to avoid the horror of watching my own child die. I never did either.

In February of the second year of my genetic fellowship, as Jimm and I strolled on a silvery beach on the Turks and Caicos Islands one night during a week's holiday, I wished for a baby on a shooting star that fell into the ocean. I had stopped taking my birth control pills earlier that month, but Jimm remained hesitant.

"Why don't we wait 'til August, after your genetics exams are done, and then we could have a spring baby," he said in April.

His was a logical plan – no nausea, no pregnancy worries as I crammed long nights for my exams. Damn it, did he always have to be right?

He wasn't this time – as he spoke those words, Jack was already a three-week-old embryo burrowing into the lining of my uterus. Come May, as I waited for my period so that I could restart my birth control pills, I was too busy cramming for my written exam to realize that it was late.

I had requested a week's vacation before the exam to study and review.

On the Tuesday of that week, I felt nauseated when I woke up. I wondered if I had eaten something wonky the night before, but the feeling passed. I did not mention it to Jimm, but the next morning the nausea returned. This time, too, it lasted less than a minute.

On the Thursday – no waking up to nausea – I crawled out of bed early to get a head start on revisions. Textbooks, medical atlases and notes were stacked on my dining table. I brewed a cup of coffee, Polish-style – boiling water poured into a large ceramic mug over two heaping tablespoons of freshly ground coffee. As the brew cooled, the grounds sank and the liquid acquired a muddy, viscous consistency. I always drank it black, bitingly bitter.

I thudded the mug next to *Gorlin's Syndromes of the Head and Neck*, a three-pound brick of a compendium, and studied. After about an hour, I realized that I had sipped the coffee only once and that the coffee in the mug next to my elbow had cooled to a tepid murk. I stared at it for a moment, nonplussed – I always gulped my coffee hot – and shuffled to the kitchen to brew another. An hour later, another mug of coffee had cooled on the table.

I don't know what made me pull out the pregnancy test left from a scare a few years earlier. I checked the expiry date – it was still valid. Warm urine splashed over my fingers before the stream hit the stick. I washed my hands and lifted the stick to my eyes and squinted – I had left my glasses on the living room table. The liquid front was slowly advancing across the paper stick. As it hit the testing area, a thick, navy-blue line popped up almost instantly. There was no mistaking its presence. My heart rate doubled.

Must be the control strip, I thought. It had changed so quickly.

As a second, ghostly blue line appeared more slowly, I read the instructions – the thin line was the control. The thick, heavy one that had appeared so fast, so exuberantly, was the positive result. My positive pregnancy test result. I was pregnant.

I didn't want to tell Jimm over the phone. He was scheduled to moonlight at Toronto East General emergency that night, starting at 6:00 p.m., so I had to wait. I couldn't concentrate on my books. I couldn't tell anyone, either – Jimm should hear the news first.

Finally, at about five in the afternoon, I phoned for a taxi. The cabbie pulled up in an orange-and-teal Beck Taxi. He was a chubby throwback to the hippie era, his shaggy grey hair tied in a ponytail. Chatty.

"You work there at the hospital?" he asked.

"My husband does. I'm on my way to tell him that I am pregnant," I blurted out. I would never see this man again, so it did not matter that he knew before Jimm.

"Congratulations!" he shouted and tapped the horn with his gnarled hand.

✒

I found Jimm elbow-deep in charts. He had just gotten a handover from the day shift and had that distracted look he sported whenever he concentrated on work.

"I need to talk to you," I said. "Now," I added, when his eyes swung toward the stack of charts.

In the dingy elevator rising two floors up to his call room, I thrust the pregnancy test at him and watched his face. I couldn't even wait to get to the privacy of his on-call room.

"What ..." His eyes flashed across the plastic wand, then to my face. He grinned.

"I'm pregnant. We're going to have a baby!"

✒

And then I went and told everybody.

I did not know one was supposed to wait until twelve weeks or until after the ultrasound; I did not know the Canadian norms about what to say to whom. I told everybody, whether they wanted to listen or not. Once I gushed to a pediatric resident colleague for a good ten minutes, only to find the following week from somebody else that she, too, was pregnant. I felt betrayed – why hadn't she told me? But she probably could not get a word in edgewise. Another time, after I enthused how easily I had gotten pregnant – I think I uttered my favourite line: "I just sneezed" – a woman, her face an angry shade of puce, regaled me with a nail-biting account of her five pregnancy losses and a drawn-out saga of artificial insemination.

"How far along is she?" I overheard one of the female geneticists ask Joe that first luminous week.

"Probably two weeks," Joe said, and the woman snickered. Yes, it would be like me to tell everybody the moment it happened. Heck, I did tell everybody the moment it happened.

I didn't care. I was having a baby.

But I still had to pass my genetics fellowship exams, a certification by the Canadian College of Medical Geneticists. I wrote the multiple-choice and essay exams the week after I found out I was pregnant, and then I realized that I could not study any more genetics until after I had my prenatal ultrasound and the maternal serum screening results in hand. That was almost three months away, but I didn't care – I had to know that my baby was okay before I could study all the ways in which a pregnancy could go wrong.

When I was a medical student, in the mid-'80s, it was discovered that women who carried fetuses with Down syndrome had a very low level of a pregnancy-related protein called alpha-fetoprotein. This protein, a fetal form of albumin, which is a major component of human blood, seeped through the placenta into the mother's bloodstream where it could be easily measured. Suddenly, there was a method to screen for Down syndrome during pregnancy without the need for the invasive amniocentesis. When I read about it for the first time, I thought it was brilliant: I would not have to worry about having a baby with Down syndrome. At the time, I was terrified of having a child with an intellectual disability.

In 1994, when I became a fellow in genetics, the addition of a measurement of two other markers in the mother's blood further improved Down syndrome screening. Called "maternal serum screening," in addition to looking for Down syndrome the blood test also screened for trisomy 18 and 13 (two conditions similar to Down syndrome in that they result from a triplication of a chromosome, but different in that they cause much more profound intellectual disability and severe birth defects; these babies seldom survived beyond the newborn period). Some arcane statistical methods combined the blood test results with the mother's age – because the older the mother, the higher the risk of a chromosomal anomaly – and arrived at a combined risk of having a baby with one of the trisomies. If the risk was high enough, a woman had the option to test the baby's chromosomes directly: she could have an amniocentesis.

At that time, it was also recognized that a thickening of the skin at the nape of the fetus's neck could sometimes signal the presence of chromosomal anomalies such as Turner syndrome (which affected only girls) and Down syndrome. In the upcoming years, the fetal nuchal thickness measurement would become part of the integrated screening that further narrowed down the risks of a chromosomal abnormality. In the mid-'90s, a nuchal fold measurement and maternal serum screening were offered to all pregnant women while amniocentesis was reserved for women who were thirty-five or older, or who had a positive screening test.

Thus, during my first pregnancy, my age – thirty-two years old at the time of delivery – did not qualify me for an amniocentesis. A woman of that age has a 1:769 risk of having a baby with Down syndrome, thus my chances were too low to risk an amniocentesis, which has a one in two hundred risk of a miscarriage. Instead, I had the screening tests – the blood measurements and a detailed ultrasound. My obstetrician would probably have supported me had I requested an amniocentesis – "maternal anxiety" was the routine reason given in such situations – but I believed in the science behind the screening test.

My screen was negative – it reduced my risk of having a baby with Down syndrome to one in fifteen thousand, that of a fifteen-year-old. Because it is not a diagnostic test, the result of a screen test is never reported as zero but only as a probability. There was only the ultrasound left and then I could enjoy my pregnancy. Not that I wasn't enjoying it already – I loved being pregnant. I had no nausea, no vomiting; only overwhelming fatigue slowed me down. In the past, I would run up the stairs at St. Patrick Station; now I rode the escalator up from the train platform every morning on the way to work. But I didn't care about that.

Come July, at eighteen weeks of pregnancy, I went for my ultrasound alone – Jimm was working in Hamilton, busy with his clinical duties and research. We decided that I would be fine by myself. I was a genetics fellow; I knew the hospital and what to expect. I would be fine.

Jimm and I had discussed if we wanted to know the sex of the baby, and in the end we decided that we did not. I practised saying, "No, let's just make sure that everything is okay and maybe at the end I'll ask."

I repeated that phrase as I walked under the hissing fluorescent lights of the corridor on the first floor of Norman Urquhart Wing at Toronto General Hospital, five floors below David's office: "No, let's just make sure that everything is okay and then I'll decide." Please, let everything be okay.

I remember that I was wearing Jimm's pants. By that time, all mine had become too tight for my thickening waist, and he had a lovely pair of summer wool slacks in tiny black-and-white houndstooth check, which I requisitioned. The tech ushered me into a curtained, semi-dark cubicle where I slipped them down my belly and lifted my shirt.

"This is going to be cold," the tech said as she squirted a blue-green gel onto my skin, which goose-pimpled instantly. She touched the crystal of the probe just above my pubic hair and adjusted a dial under the computer screen.

"Do you want to know the sex of the baby?" she asked.

"No, let's just make sure that everything is okay and then I'll decide." It came out properly, even though my voice was shaking.

She should have left it at that. Instead, she said, "Because I know already."

So, it's a boy, I thought. Joy flooded me – I always wanted to have a boy for my firstborn.

"It's a boy," I blurted out, and she whirled around and faced me. I shrugged. "Only if you see the penis floating around can you be so sure so quickly." I did know that much.

"Are you a nurse?" she asked.

"I'm a genetics fellow," I said. "I've worked with David Chitayat, upstairs."

Maybe I imagined her discomfort as she turned back to the screen.

As she continued the scan, I craned my neck to see the screen better. A butterfly-shaped movement, rapid and fluttery, was the heart. An arm topped with a broomstick of hand bones flitted by. The zipper of the spine, the vertebrae aligned along a smooth curve. And then a circular grey shadow, a cross-section I did not recognize, the tech's callipers marking a lighter, curvier line at the bottom of the screen.

"What are you measuring?" I asked.

"The nuchal fold," she answered without moving her eyes from the screen.

My heart stopped. I know it did not, but it felt like it did. My baby boy was going to have Down syndrome. I was going to have a baby with Down syndrome.

Sweat can pour out of your skin in the blink of an eye. A puddle collected between my breasts and my armpits were dripping; my panties were soaked as sweat pooled in my groin. Wetness spread in the crooks of my elbows and behind my ears, where it mixed with the tears flowing soundlessly down my temples. They turned freezing cold, but I kept quiet. I was not going to cry because if I did, I would howl like a wounded wolf.

"How ... how thick is the nuchal?" I finally choked out.

"I don't remember," the tech said, her eyes still on the screen. I finally let out a sound – a stifled groan, a mourning for all my hopes and dreams. Her face snapped toward me.

"What's wrong?" Her wrist flopped and the probe on my belly lost contact with the skin – the screen went black.

"The baby, my baby, has Down syndrome ..."

"What? How ...?" Her voice rose with every word.

"You measured the nuchal," I sobbed. "It's thickened, so that means it's Down's because it's a boy."

"No! We measure it on everybody. Don't you know that?"

I did not. I thought they would only measure it if it was obviously thickened.

"You do?" I breathed, not ready to believe her yet.

"The nuchal wasn't thickened at all," she said.

I wiped the tears from my cheeks with the backs of my hands. She brought me green surgical towels and I mopped the sweat from between and under my breasts, and from the nape – the nape! – and front of my neck. I dried my face. She gave me a paper cup with ice water. I drained it in three gulps.

"Okay," I said. "No Down syndrome."

She finished the scan and brought in the radiologist to review the images. When I told him what had happened, he only said, "If we didn't measure it on everybody, we wouldn't know what's normal." He barely glanced at me as he gave my baby a pass and left the room.

I staggered out of the radiology department and found a pay phone in the hallway and paged Jimm out of his ward rounds at McMaster.

"Jimm, it's Jack!" I blurted into the receiver.

"What?"

"My ultrasound? It's a boy." I didn't tell him about the Down syndrome.

"That's wonderful," he said, but he had to get back to rounds. "We'll talk about it tonight," he said and hung up. I stared at the buttons of the pay phone for a bit, then placed the receiver into its cradle. My baby boy was fine.

✒

What if it had not been a misunderstanding? What if the nuchal fold had been thickened, and the amniocentesis – which I know I would have had – had shown an extra chromosome 21? By the time the results would have arrived, I would have not only seen Jack on the ultrasound but also felt him move deep inside me. I would have shared my body with him for twenty-one or twenty-two weeks. I had already watched the two little lines of his heartbeat tapping together at a speed too rapid to comprehend during that very first ultrasound at six weeks. I had been talking to him from that moment in the bathroom when the blue line appeared. Would I have stopped the pregnancy? Most likely.

Four and a half years later, pregnant with my second son and, at thirty-five, old enough for chromosome analysis, I chose chorionic villus sampling, an analysis of the baby's chromosomes from a tiny fragment of the placenta that's obtained at twelve weeks of pregnancy, much earlier than an amniocentesis. It has a slightly higher risk of miscarriage than amniocentesis, but if I had to stop nobody would have been the wiser – my pregnancy would not have shown yet. So yes, again, I thought about stopping.

How would I have fared if I'd had a child with a disability? I think I could have coped with a child with a physical disability or with a life-shortening condition. It was the autism-intellectual disability spectrum that I felt would have destroyed me – the child that did not recognize you, that did not give back in love or smiles or hugs, the child oblivious to your presence and love and devotion. The child that would dart out naked into the middle of traffic, physically able to run, open doors, jump down stairs with no comprehension of danger. A child with Down syndrome could sit at the table at Red Lobster and share their crab leg with a stranger at the next table, but a girl with Cornelia de Lange syndrome who bit the top of her hand to the point of needing stitches – yes, she went straight from my clinic to emergency – was altogether different.

I did not want to have a child with any type of intellectual disability. My mental prowess, my mind, however flawed, was my identity and I wanted the same for my children.

➡

Three weeks after my ultrasound, on Friday morning teaching rounds, one of the residents presented a case of a boy with pyruvate decarboxylase deficiency, a deadly metabolic disease in which the cells are unable to utilize glucose for energy – essentially, they starve to death in the face of plenty. Since the brain is the most energy-guzzling organ in the body, these boys have severe brain damage. And since pyruvate decarboxylase is encoded on the X chromosome, only boys get this disease. The X chromosome is much larger than the male-determining Y, therefore if a boy receives from his mother an X chromosome with a mutation, it will cause disease. A woman who carries the mutation is not affected because she has another, normally functioning X chromosome; many such women do not know that they are carriers until they have an affected son.

In the conference room, we segued into a discussion of X-linked inheritance, and suddenly I realized that now, knowing that I was carrying a boy, I had a whole new class of genetic diseases to worry about. Muscular dystrophy, Lesch-Nyhan syndrome, Hunter disease – a laundry list of horrible disorders, diseases and deficiencies that might affect my baby son scrolled through my brain. Fear grabbed me.

Yet somehow, I managed to shake it off. "I'll think about it later," I thought. "I can't be thinking about it, it will drive me crazy." I pushed all these dreadful possibilities out of my mind. There was no point worrying about them. They might never happen. They were not real. Somehow, I managed to stave off the physician mother syndrome, the more mature version of medical student syndrome.

Now that my screening reported a low risk for Down syndrome and other trisomies, and the ultrasound showed no major birth defects, I had to begin reviewing those and other genetic conditions for my fellowship exam. It was scheduled for September and I had no time to waste. I hit the books again to prepare for the oral part of the genetics fellowship exam. And that was when I realized that I could not bear to look at a photo of a baby with harlequin-type ichthyosis in my *Diagnostic Dysmorphology* textbook. I had seen the photo many times before as I read and reread the text, and it did not cause any disquiet. But one day, as I was reviewing the lists of dysmorphic features, the photo ambushed me. I had seen a real newborn with this condition in the SickKids NICU the previous year, the baby pumped full of morphine to dull the pain of the deeply cracked skin peeling off his body, his crimson lips and eyelids extruded between the armour-hard scales of his face. Now, the black-and-white photo took my breath away. No, I didn't cut up the book like my mother had done with the *Little Encyclopedia*, but I stuck several yellow Post-it Notes over the black-and-white photo and secured them with paper clips so that they wouldn't accidentally fly off as I turned the pages. It remained covered until well after my son's birth, when imagining the pain the little one must have suffered became a bit more bearable.

✒

Jack was born at St. Michael's Hospital after a fifteen-hour train-wreck of a labour. At one moment in the delivery room, the pain was such that I actually considered jumping out the fourth-storey window, but all windows on the labour floor were secured shut. My epidural didn't work well, and even though paralyzed from the waist down from all the anaesthetic top-ups, with every contraction I felt like I was being torn in half lengthwise, from the crotch up. Jack's head would not rotate in the birth canal and he was coming out face-up, the shelf on the back of his head pressing on my sacrum and tailbone. In the end, I was wheeled into the operating room. "We have to do a mid-forceps rotation," the obstetrician said. "If that doesn't work, I'll have to section you." I didn't care if I was going to end up with a Caesarean – I just wanted the pain to stop.

They finally managed to extract Jack after an episiotomy cut that felt like it stretched from my groin to my right ear and after twisting him inside me. He emerged without a drop of blood on him and with a perfectly round head. Jimm wouldn't hold him when the nurse handed Jack to him. "Margaret did all the work, she should hold him first," he said, and my heart swelled with love for him. But all the doses of anaesthetic I had received extended the paralysis up to my chest and the nurse worried that I would drop the baby. Only after all the stitches went in and some of the anaesthesia wore off was I able to stare into the huge blue eyes of my son. He stared right back, his eyes clear and fully focused. It was as if we had known each other forever. His head was round, unmoulded by the delivery, fuzzed with the faintest, blondish red hair.

With that first glimpse, his features etched themselves onto my retinas, never to be erased – I can still see him as that minutes-old newborn. Round pink cheeks; pouty and full lips the colour of poppies; tiny, flat pink shells of ears. Silky fingers with pearls of the most darling fingernails. Joy swept over me like a huge ocean wave and took hold of every last molecule of my body; selfless love and radiant delight like I had never experienced brought me to my knees. The rational, sceptical, occasionally cynical me was defeated in a flash by a mother's love for her child.

My parents and my sister visited us that first evening. For years, my parents never said anything about a grandchild, never inquired whether Jimm and I would be getting pregnant. Even my mother showed remarkable restraint and never hinted that there must be something wrong with me.

Only when Jack was a few months old did she tell me that all of their Polish friends had been noseying as to why I wasn't pregnant yet. "Far be it from me to tell two doctors how to make a baby" was my father's response to all of their enquires.

☞

As the high of the delivery wore off, the first weeks of life with Jack became a blur of exhaustion punctuated by moments of panic. The first occurred while still in the hospital when, on his second day of life, his temperature plummeted, his face paled, and his fingers and toes turned blue. The pediatrician ordered X-rays to look for pneumonia or a heart defect, and blood and urine tests for infection. I frantically tried to page Jimm through the hospital operator who would not put through a long-distance call to Hamilton for me. I tried calling my friends but got so flummoxed I couldn't remember Raymond's or Mannie's numbers; Lynn was doing a cardiology fellowship in Ann Arbor by that time. I didn't want to worry my parents, so I was all alone in my terror staring at the plastic incubator with my firstborn splayed with an oxygen probe on his tiny foot and a temperature monitor on his chest. All my studying, all my training, and I was helpless to do anything for him except list all the terrible things that could be wrong. I couldn't even touch him – he needed to stay warm, and with every opening of the incubator's hatches, his temperature dropped. With my belly hanging out as if I were still pregnant, my feet swollen into two pillows from all the intravenous fluid they had pumped into me the day before, I paced, sore-crotched, in the hallway outside the nursery. I think that I didn't dissolve into a puddle of anguish only because the delivery endorphins and oxytocin were still kicking around my system. A few hours later, Jack pinked up, and when the nurse handed him to me, all bundled up, he latched hungrily onto my breast. Preliminary tests all came back normal, so by the time Jimm returned from Hamilton, I was able to reassure him that everything was all right. He never knew how terrified I had been – all he saw was a healthy pink son at my breast.

At home, we soon established a routine – I paced in our two-bedroom apartment from the living room to the bedroom while Jack slept or cried, fed and pooped. The days flew by as I changed diapers and breastfed him on demand. When he napped, instead of resting, I foolishly wrote two case reports and prepared them for publication. It never occurred to me that I could nap when he did, and no one gave me that advice. At the time, submissions to medical journals were all done on paper; the manuscript and the accompanying photographs – in triplicate – were sent by post. Brain muddled with fatigue, I glued tiny labels on the backs of the black-and-white photos, marking the top of each with an arrow and hand-printing my name in pencil as specified by the submission guidelines. When Jimm arrived home in the evening after his commute from Hamilton, I was half-crazed with exhaustion, but I had never been happier: I had given birth to a beautiful, healthy boy, and I was so proud of him and myself.

Entirely of his own volition, from the day we brought Jack home, Jimm had decided that I should pump milk and allow him to bottle-feed Jack every other night so that I could get some sleep. He stuck to his plan, his work and research and commuting notwithstanding. The nights when it was my turn to get up, I breastfed in the rocking chair reading *Star Trek* paperbacks Jimm kept buying for me and terrifying myself with the dysmorphic features that I noticed in Jack.

On the back flap of Jack's milestones book lives a list of physical findings that I had thought were wrong with him during the first seven months of his life. At one point or another – usually in the middle of the night but not always – I had thought that he had dysplastic (abnormal) ears, natal teeth, a proximally set thumb (too close to the wrist), abnormally wrinkled skin on his soles, bitemporal narrowing (his forehead was too narrow), flat forehead with absent brow ridges and epicanthal folds (folds of skin covering the inner corners of his eyes). As if that wasn't enough, there were also moments of insanity when I believed that he had Beckwith-Wiedemann syndrome because he gained weight very fast, even though he did not get any formula, and because he stuck out his tongue – definite macroglossia (enlarged tongue); or an infiltrating malignant tumour (cancer) of his tongue, which turned out to be a Candida infection; or glycogen storage disease type 1, because he sweated a lot at night; or stomach reflux. None of those were true, of course, but by the time he was six weeks old, I had managed to corral the top dermatologist and the top ophthalmologist at SickKids to check him out. Both Bernice Krafchik and Alex Levine were understanding if – justifiably – amused. Yes, he had anisocoria – uneven pupils – but it was within normal limits, and the tiny burst vessels on his cheeks were not a sign of impending liver failure. I can joke now about all this, but my fears for his health and safety overwhelmed me almost every night. Come daylight, I was able to see his toes and tongue and eyes and fingers for what they were: normal and adorable.

The most terrifying moment was when, for a harrowing half-hour, I believed that Jack had Lesch-Nyhan syndrome, a dreadful disease of intellectual disability and lack of pain sensation that led the boys with it (it only affected boys, it was an X-linked condition) to chew away their lips, tongue, fingers and whatever other body part they were able to reach with their teeth, tearing flesh away and gouging out wounds. I had learned about this horrific condition when I first worked with Joe Clarke. Its gruesomeness both scared and repelled me.

What mother worries about Lesch-Nyhan syndrome when her baby son wiggles his bum as he learns to coordinate his legs and trunk while on his tummy? It was because his diapers were stained pink. Uric acid is a common breakdown product in the human body and its bright pink crystals can appear in diapers when babies are even slightly dehydrated. But I knew that boys with Lesch-Nyhan syndrome excrete huge amounts of uric acid, so of course Jack, with the tiny mauve splotches in his pee, had to have it. At least that's what I thought when I read a case report where an affected boy had presented with wriggling of his legs being the first sign of Lesch-Nyhan syndrome. With this realization, I became one big pounding, terrified heart – I felt my pulse in my belly, chest, fingertips as fear, or rather adrenaline, coursed through me. Adrenaline, the hormone of fear, of the atavistic fight-or-flight response – but if Jack had a terrible disease, I couldn't outrun it. I couldn't fight it. I would simply freeze and collapse.

Of course, Jack did not have Lesch-Nyhan syndrome, but I needed

David Chitayat to reassure me of that. He gently and kindly talked me off the ledge when I paged him that afternoon.

☞

In September 1996, I passed my qualifying oral exams in genetics while six months pregnant. Since a job offer at SickKids was not forthcoming, I had to consider other options. At the time, no academic centre in Canada needed a metabolic specialist, but the university hospitals in Vancouver, Edmonton and Hamilton were advertising positions for a clinical geneticist. I wanted to work exclusively as a metabolics consultant, like Joe Clarke, but I wanted – no, needed – a job more, so I applied to all three. By then, Jimm had been commuting to Hamilton from Toronto for four years and I promised both of us that I would take a job anywhere as long as he would not have to do that commute anymore – he had done enough sacrificing. Hamilton, where he already had a clinical scholar position, an entry point without a university appointment, was an obvious choice. But the offer from McMaster did not come even after two rounds of interviews. I became despondent: fifteen years of post-secondary education, a babe in arms and no job in sight, I applied for the two jobs in Western Canada.

In the middle of April, Jimm and I packed up our son, his car seat, his stroller, the diaper bag and the breast pump, and the three of us flew west for interviews in Edmonton and Vancouver. There were no positions for an academic internist for Jimm at either, but we thought that we had to at least check out the jobs for me. We ruled out Edmonton the day after we landed, when the thermometer dropped to minus eighteen degrees centigrade – it was just too damn cold. The following day, Vancouver greeted us awash in blooming magnolias, lawns scattered with daffodils and primroses. Aaaah, warmth.

McMaster finally came through with a job offer, but I had one more thing to do before I accepted it. I knocked on the door to Joe's office. Back in the fall, when I had begun to look for a job, he had requested that I speak to him before accepting any offers. He invited me in, closed the door and told me that I had a job at SickKids if I wanted it.

If I wanted it?! For years this had been my driving force, my guiding light, my unicorn: a staff position at the hallowed halls of the Hospital for Sick Children in Toronto. Finally, I thought, after all these years of hinting at how much I wanted to work there. Wait, what? He had known that I travelled across the country for interviews while breastfeeding an infant yet he never said a word?

To my questions about the details of the position, Joe's answers were evasive. There was to be no academic appointment – it would come if I "showed that I deserved it." There was no security: it was a contract position, renewable every year. "I also have a contract position," he said, trying to convince me as if it were the same thing. He couldn't tell me about benefits, holidays, funding for conferences and education – all spelled out in my McMaster offer.

After I left his office, I sat in the fellows' room thinking for a bit. Then I phoned Jimm, we talked briefly, and exactly twenty-one minutes later I accepted McMaster University's offer.

Part Two

Treatments & Remedies

7

Our little family moved to Hamilton in the early summer of 1997. Jimm found a house within walking distance to the university and I agreed, house unseen. (If I couldn't trust him with finding us a good home, how could I trust him with our life?) It was a two-storey, three-bedroom brick house with neglected back and front lawns, the backyard surrounded by a hedge while a tall maple shaded the front. We rented because we truly believed that we would not be staying in Hamilton for more than two or three years; Jimm has always wanted to go back to Toronto, his hometown, and neither of us relished being banished to the medical backwaters of Hamilton, as we thought of it then. That May, I found Jack a spot in a daycare associated with the Early Childhood Education program at the local community college and paid for it right away – such places were hard to come by.

The first day of my real job, August 1, was a Friday. By late morning, I already had four consults in the NICU. When I arrived at the nursery, a two-room unit crammed full of incubators and whooshing ventilators and pinging intravenous pumps, the NICU chief told me that they had been waiting for the "real geneticist" for a while. A compliment but also a tremendous responsibility – what if I couldn't deliver? One of the patients I saw that day was a fourteen-week-old boy with shortened limbs who was still in the nursery because of severe feeding difficulties. I tentatively diagnosed him as having spondylometaphyseal dysplasia and was thrilled when, a week later, a consultant from the Cedars-Sinai Skeletal Dysplasia Registry confirmed my impression – I had couriered the boy's X-rays to Los Angeles for a second opinion.

☞

During my job interviews at McMaster, I had been told that 50 percent of my salary would originate from the provincial Maternal Serum Screening

Program. The head of the prenatal service made it clear that he expected me to provide a corresponding proportion of clinical service as a consultant in prenatal genetics. That had given me pause: after all, prenatal was the subspecialty I liked the least and never wanted to have much to do with. But I needed a job. And Jimm had always wanted to study blood clots and their disorders, and McMaster had an international reputation in this field. I accepted the position, and I took this part of the job seriously.

One of the first challenges was navigating the relationship between me, as a staff physician, and the genetic counsellors. Genetic counsellors counsel patients and families on diagnosed diseases, determine the family history of such conditions and provide psychological support to affected individuals and their family members. They explain in simple terms the intricacies of the genetic code and the biological principles underlying human inheritance the way Hunt Willard had us do in our medical school genetics course. But the final and ultimate responsibility for the correct diagnosis and counselling lies with the physician who sees the patients, no matter how briefly. The only patients who see a geneticist first are those who require a diagnostic assessment for as-yet undiagnosed conditions. At that time at McMaster there were only three full-time counsellors: Susan and Tim in clinical genetics, and Marlene in prenatal diagnosis. During my training at SickKids, I always felt that I would never match a counsellor's confidence, either as a fellow or a staff physician. Frankly, I was afraid of them – they were all excellent professionals and great at their job, but they bossed around the fellows and residents mercilessly. Some were less than collegial. Once, a genetic counsellor paged me twice in three minutes while I was in a sterile hood trying to set up a DNA experiment during my research rotation. I had to strip my sterile gown, mask and gloves to phone her. She wanted to know about a patient I had seen the week before.

"It's all in the chart," I told her. "Didn't you see it?"

"I haven't looked for the chart," she said sanguinely. I knew that the chart was in the filing cabinet directly outside her office and yet I said nothing. Counsellors were permanent staff while we fellows changed every year and were expendable – it didn't pay to piss them off. Every day, I bit my tongue and watched my step because I wanted that dream job at SickKids. At work, I let them walk all over me and stewed in private, waiting for the day when I would become a staff physician. Then they would stop, I thought, even if David Chitayat had warned me that "they will always treat you like a fellow if you get a job at the place where you trained." Since my SickKids job never materialized, I couldn't test his theory, but I suspect he was right.

What I didn't realize during my training but have since learned in spades was that genetic counsellors were put on this earth to keep clinical geneticists out of trouble – so many times a counsellor's timely suggestion saved the day, and my ass. Genetic counsellors have a Master of Science in – you guessed it – genetic counselling, which is preceded by at least a Bachelor of Science in genetics or human biology. I am convinced that the counselling training programs choose their candidates for their intelligence, confidence and assertiveness, and my genetics fellow colleagues agreed, especially with the assertiveness part. Counsellors do not fear speaking their mind.

The counsellor's job is demanding and draining and difficult. Before they – or I – see a patient, they research the available information across the vastness of genetic knowledge. They find the appropriate genetic tests and procure educational materials for the patients and their families. During counselling sessions – which sometimes take up to two hours – they document generations of family history and explain complex genetic concepts in layman's terms. Then they write detailed consult letters, which I read and co-sign. Every day, genetic counsellors give abnormal genetic tests results, either on the phone in the case of time-sensitive prenatal tests or in person, in clinic, the geneticists playing second fiddle to their expertise in explaining genetic concepts. They field tearful and angry phone calls from parents and patients, and provide emotional support following a difficult diagnosis; they arrange follow-ups with social workers and with other consultants. They are the buffer around the awfulness of prenatal and clinical genetics. I could never do my job without genetic counsellors.

☞

I enjoyed working at McMaster from day one. The older pediatricians – almost all middle-aged white men; there was only one female attending neonatologist in the NICU – were welcoming and affable while my peers in the other specialities were simply nice people. Some of the younger ones were also veterans of training programs at SickKids but there was none of its cutthroat undercurrent. At the time, McMaster Children's Hospital, housed in the adult McMaster University Hospital, was comprised of two in-patient wards, four dedicated pediatric beds in the adult ICU and the three levels of newborn nurseries, including the largest NICU in the province. And while I revelled in the low-key and friendly climate, I missed the cutting-edge academia and genetics research for which SickKids was famous. Compared to what I had experienced in Toronto, McMaster felt like a genetics backwater. Even the McMaster University Medical Centre – a brutalist '70s-style bunker with a sunless central courtyard, and cracked and stained grey concrete – was in desolate contrast to the brand-new, airy, spacious SickKids Atrium I had left behind.

I shared the clinical and metabolic service with Dr. Don Whelan, a pediatrician nearing retirement, who single-handedly had been providing all of the genetic, prenatal and metabolic consultations at McMaster for almost a decade. Don was available to answer any questions I had, but in reality, the years of teachers and instructors overseeing my actions were over. There was no more safety net. Now, I alone was responsible – medically, morally and legally – for making the right diagnosis and managing a patient's care correctly. After the relative security of my residency and fellowship years, the time had come for me to take off the training wheels.

Nowhere was my transformation more poignant and demanding than in prenatal genetics. Prenatal diagnosis truly is a matter of life and death. Termination of pregnancy is the only treatment available for the vast majority of genetic diseases, but only if they are detected early enough. Even though parents make the final decision, their deliberations depend on my interpretation and how I present the facts during counselling. Because

I had not been interested in prenatal genetics during my fellowship, once I was hired at McMaster, I threw myself into learning it. I read papers and studied textbooks, and, as usual, covered pads of paper with notes. At the American Society of Human Genetics meeting in Baltimore that year, I signed up for a four-hour workshop on the diagnostic investigations of pregnancy demise and stillbirth. I promised myself that I would care for the pregnant patients in Hamilton as well as David did for his in Toronto.

At McMaster, I did not consult on all patients with positive prenatal screening results because there were too many of them. The obstetricians supervised the one genetic counsellor and the genetic nurse for those cases. For many years, before more counsellors were hired in the Prenatal Diagnosis clinic, Marlene took the brunt of the difficult prenatal cases. She was the one to tell parents the extent of the anomalies found on an ultrasound, their significance, their severity. Anencephaly, spina bifida, missing limbs, cleft lip, heart defects – she has seen it all and worse. But complex chromosomal anomalies and fetuses with multiple birth defects discovered during routine ultrasounds were my responsibility. "We save the hard cases for you," Marlene quipped once, but it was no joke. I crawled up a very steep learning curve those first few months on the job.

As in metabolics, I loved putting together the pieces of the puzzle and arriving at a diagnosis, except now the clues arrived as shadowy images of extra fingers and toes, or malformed brains in various combinations and permutations: missing cerebellum and cleft upper lip, suggestive of oro-facial-digital syndrome type I (there are six others); tiny, undergrown baby with lemon-shaped skull and clenched fingers, possible trisomy 18. The hunt was on. I was chasing zebras again – and I realized, with surprise, that I was enjoying the prenatal diagnosis service. For some of the conditions there were tests to confirm my clinical diagnosis, but for many all I had was my training and knowledge.

Sometimes my excitement at diagnosing got the better of me. Once, I blurted out to the parents of a boy with hand and foot anomalies, "Fingers and toes everywhere!" A nurse had said that to me while I examined him during my consultation and I repeated the phrase without thinking when

I ran into his parents outside the NICU. I had just returned from Toronto, thrilled that David had confirmed my diagnosis of acrocallosal syndrome in their baby, a diagnosis I had been searching for since I first saw seven toes on the boy's left foot and eight on the right, in addition to his extra pinkies and duplicated thumbs, during the twenty-week ultrasound. The father blanched. Even as the words were leaving my mouth, I could not believe what I was saying. I apologized immediately. Later, I learned that the father had been demanding all along that Warren wear mittens even in the heat of summer, so that nobody would see his extra digits.

I have never since done anything that thoughtless or inconsiderate.

But I was enjoying more than the diagnostic challenges. Maybe it was because these patients and their parents were finally my responsibility, maybe it was because I had been through a pregnancy and birth myself, but something had shifted in my attitude toward prenatal genetics. I cared about the mothers and their partners sitting across the table from me more deeply and differently than I had ever cared about any of my patients before. The enormity of the situation was not lost on me – these parents were making decisions about their children's lives based on the diagnoses I made and on my counselling. Soon I realized that I could be gentle and warm even under the direst of circumstances. Marlene and, later, other genetic counsellors, as well as prenatal social workers, complimented me on my counselling and people skills. Sometimes, to my surprise, parents smiled when they saw me again, even if previously I had given them terrible news. And I really looked forward to being able to tell them the good news when the next pregnancy came along – normal test results, normal ultrasound. Those happy follow-ups kept me going and kept me sane. I had insisted on seeing them, and the genetic counsellors were happy to oblige. "Go home and enjoy the rest of your pregnancy" was my favourite phrase, always adding, "As much as any parent can enjoy the uncertainty and worry. Having kids is a marathon of worry." That always elicited a smile.

☞

More often than not, prenatal diagnosis is a race against time. We – I – had to figure out the diagnosis before the deadline for termination in Ontario had passed. In the mid-'90s, terminations could be performed at specialized centres until twenty-two weeks of pregnancy if the baby had a condition that would result in early death or severe physical or intellectual disability. After that deadline, a woman who wanted to stop a pregnancy had to be referred to a clinic in Wichita, Kansas, where Dr. George Tiller offered terminations as late as forty weeks. Yes, that's full term. He provided his services until 2009 when a pro-life activist shot him in the head in his Kansas church as Dr. Tiller handed out programs for the Sunday service, the bulletproof vest he wore every day proving useless.

Rarely would a prenatal case be easy, with a clear-cut diagnosis that equalled a clear-cut prognosis and straightforward counselling. Those cases were mainly fetuses with severe chromosomal imbalances or grave brain malformations. As I had promised myself I would do at the bedside of the baby girl with Wolf-Hirschhorn syndrome that day at SickKids, I explained as explicitly as possible: "This baby will always be in diapers, he will never learn to walk or speak," or "You will always need to look after her – she will always be like a newborn," or "He will be able to walk and run, but he won't be able to think, to control his impulses or to judge danger." Parents deserved to know the truth – no sugar-coating, no euphemisms.

Almost always, I could reassure parents that it was not their fault: "Mothers in your situation – fathers, too – look in the mirror and wonder if it was something they did to cause their baby's problems. That glass of wine? That fight you had that day? Those didn't cause it. It was a gene change that happened long before the baby was even conceived." Their shoulders would slide down their back and their faces would lose some of that doomed expression. Relief brightened their faces when I said that the chances of recurrence were 2 or 10 or 25 percent since, more often than not, they had convinced themselves that they would never have a healthy baby. "You can," I would tell them, truthfully.

☞

I examined each fetus after delivery. The first time I arrived on the hospital ward where genetic terminations were performed, I asked the charge nurse about a patient admitted for TA, short for therapeutic abortion.

"We don't call it 'TA,'" she said.

"What do we call it?" I asked, feeling inadequate and inappropriate.

"Termination of pregnancy," she answered.

Right. These were wanted, long-awaited babies whose un-started lives were cherished, whose possibility was mourned when lost.

I've lost count of how many fetuses I have examined over the past twenty-four years – about three hundred or more; about fifteen or so for each year in practice. Some were still warm when I unwrapped them from the crocheted blanket made by a volunteer, but most were cold because after delivery the nurses kept them in a small fridge in the clean utility room on the ward. I measured and weighed them, examined their bodies the way I had seen David examine that first fetus. I took photos and wrote a note on the chart detailing the baby's sex and any anomalies I observed, and then recorded the baby's measurements.

No matter how abnormal a fetus has appeared on the ultrasound, I always encourage parents to see the baby after delivery, so they know that there really was a baby and do not wonder for the rest of their lives what kind of "monster" they had conceived. Like I'd learned as a child reading about waterhead, the human imagination can be unrestrained and merciless, and will supply images of eyeless, nose-less faces with grotesque limbs or tails to fill the gaps in our knowledge. And while these are certainly possible, the vast majority of babies with genetic conditions appear more or less normal to the untrained eye. The parents who choose to hold their babies always tell me that they are glad they had the chance. For all babies, the nurses prepare a memory box – a Polaroid photo, an index card with inked impressions of feet and hands, a card with the time and date of delivery. Many parents come back asking for the memory box months later; until then, the social workers keep them safe.

If the parents are comfortable with it, I examine the babies in the mother's room, unwrap them on the hospital bed under the oblique light of the bedside lamp. The babies are dressed in tiny hats and minuscule full-length white shirts tied at the back and gathered at the neck and wrists, sewn by hospital volunteers; and wrapped in small crocheted blankets hooked by the loving hands of yet other volunteers. Sometimes, parents ask me to show them what I see when I examine their babies. So, slowly, quietly, as if the babies are sleeping, I point out the low-set ears or widely spaced eyes, and when I finish, I wrap them again in their gowns, slip their hats back on their soft heads.

"She looks so normal," the mother or the father sometimes says, a cue that they need reassurance that a mistake wasn't made. I point out the small differences, the minor anomalies, and explain their meaning to reassure the parents that, no, there has been no mistake. Or they say, "I expected so much worse." Others comment on how human the baby looks – even though a twenty-week fetus weighs less than half a pound, the weight of a large orange, it is still fully formed. Only the fused eyelids and the brilliant red hue of the skin differ from those of a fully grown newborn.

I was the sole genetic consultant to the prenatal service for eight years, until 2005. Every Tuesday, except for holidays, conferences and Christmas, I consulted on scheduled patients in the fourth-floor prenatal clinic and provided urgent consults the rest of the time. If I was on holiday or at a conference, Marlene provided the initial consultation under the supervision of the obstetrician on call. If a pregnancy termination occurred during my absence, when I returned, I would review the ultrasound images, the autopsy photographs and findings (if the baby had died), and the genetic results to puzzle the pieces together.

Straightforward cases were rare. Much more frequently, I had to deal with all shades of grey between two extremes: normal – whatever that means – on the one hand and severe intellectual or physical disability on the other. Nobody during my training ever mentioned how difficult prenatal diagnosis would be. I had to explain uncertainties to distressed parents. Sometimes, a combination of birth defects had a known association with intellectual disability, but with no certainty as to its extent – it was like trying to determine the functioning capabilities of a desktop computer based on the colour of its plastic shell. Some parents accepted the unknowns – "We will love the baby no matter what," they would say. Others could not tolerate any degree of uncertainty and stopped the pregnancy. I supported whatever decision they made. It wasn't for me to judge. They alone would have to live with their decision.

And, for a while, I managed to convince myself that I was immune to the grief and loss and the enormity of the decisions being made in the pre-natal clinic, but inside, prenatal was eating me alive.

My first month in prenatal at McMaster, a family doctor referred a woman whose fetus had shortened bones in his arms and legs. She was thirty-two weeks pregnant. I had reviewed the findings with Dr. Pat Mohide, the obstetrician in charge of the prenatal clinic, and we agreed that it was most likely achondroplasia, the most common form of dwarfism and one of the conditions that we can be quite certain of diagnosing prenatally.

"I'll have you know that I too had tiny toes when I was little," the mother said, vehemently, after I finished my counselling. "My baby's not going to be a dwarf."

I had not uttered the word "dwarf," nor had I mentioned the baby's toes. But she hadn't heard anything I did say: the baby had shortened thighbones and upper arms, his head loomed large with a bulging forehead, too much amniotic fluid surrounded him. The toes were the least of his problems. "My father has tiny toes, too," she threw her final argument at me.

Even that late in pregnancy I knew that life could be in the balance. I had heard about parents stopping a pregnancy because of achondroplasia as late as the ninth month.

"Why wasn't any of this picked up before?" she demanded. Her pretty face, framed by short, carefully styled blonde hair, flushed an angry red.

She wore a fitted cranberry-coloured maternity sweater and cream slacks, her feet in stylish Birkenstocks, so new the patent leather still shone next to her oversized leather bag that sat slumped on the floor. Her eyebrows arched elegantly above her bright blue eyes, which were expertly made-up. Those eyebrows crumpled now as she scowled at me.

She was maybe a year or two older than me, a few years further along the carefully planned trajectory of a professional woman. I knew nothing about her other than the history of her pregnancy, her ultrasound results and the fact that she was a lawyer. My imagination supplied the rest – the long nights studying as an undergraduate to get into law school, the cutthroat articling and junior partnership years, the desire to prove herself and to succeed. Prepared and polished, she fit the image of a competent, successful, professional woman. Substitute medical school and residency and it could have been me, except for the polish and confidence.

Now she would have a disabled baby.

"The bones of the limbs grow the most in the third trimester," I said. "I'm sure that the measurements were normal at the time of the eighteen-week scan. We can review those if you wish."

"And I can sue you for emotional distress," she snapped.

A baby with a disability clearly did not fit her life plan. It seemed I had no right to destroy her carefully constructed reality. I offered a convenient target for her anger.

I knew I was right; hers was not a complicated case or a diagnostic challenge. I did not cause the baby's genetic condition nor did I cause her emotional distress on purpose. I knew that I had delivered the facts compassionately and professionally. I did not relish the fact that the baby would have a skeletal dysplasia, but I knew that she would have to eventually believe me once her baby was born. And I realized that I was getting angry myself. Not because of her threat to report me to the College of Physicians and Surgeons but because she never said anything about her baby – it was as if her anger at me had blotted out all love and softness, all concern for the child she carried. I realized that I worried about her baby's future a lot more than I worried about my professional one.

Although I was young and inexperienced, I did recognize her fear, pure and unadulterated. But she probably would have reacted like a stepped-on snake had I named that fear; would have flailed at any expression of compassion or concern. She pretended she did not need it, she would not accept it, and all I could was slink out of the room.

Many other parents have lashed out at me, but she stands out vividly. Because she was one of my first? Because I could see some of myself in her? Perhaps. But, unlike her, I knew how wrong things could go with an embryo as it struggled to make itself whole during those first ten weeks of organ formation, totally at the mercy of its genes and environment. During my pregnancy with Jack, I never took anything for granted until I held him. Yet here was a woman who expected everything to go perfectly and who shot the messenger when it did not.

I never expected things to go right for me. Ever. Would I have reacted this way if it were my baby, if I had found out that my son was destined to be a little person? I like to think that I would respond with sadness and love, that I would have bawled my eyes out and then dealt with it. I like to think I would not threaten the physician who bore the bad news. Do I know that for sure? My pregnancy had been a dream and at home, my beautiful, fat, nine-month-old Jack crawled up my kitchen cabinets, learning to stand.

I never saw the boy when he was born – his mother refused a genetic consult after his delivery. But a few years later, I did see him at Jack's summer camp where he rolled around on the turf waiting for his mother to pick him up at the end of the day. Two years ago, I jogged past him – a young man with achondroplasia – walking with his mother on a leafy gravel trail behind my house.

☞

Another pregnant woman accused me of "wanting to kill" her baby. I recoiled as if she'd slapped me. The baby – a twenty-three-week female fetus – had hydrops fetalis, a condition in which excessive fluid accumulates under the baby's skin and in all of the abdominal and chest cavities. Such a huge amount of extra fluid in the body overwhelmed the baby's heart, which would frequently fail and cause the baby to die either in utero or shortly after birth. Hydrops is often caused by a chromosomal anomaly and I had suggested an amniocentesis to the mother. Genetic testing would not help this baby – the hydrops was far too advanced – but I needed a diagnosis to determine the chances of recurrence in the woman's next pregnancy. That was when she blurted those horrible words. Yes, I had told her that the baby was unlikely to survive given how much fluid had accumulated in her belly and chest and under her skin and around her heart but no! I did not want to kill anybody. My eyes popped wide open. I had not even mentioned a termination; I had only told her how sick her baby was.

I never pondered the moral and ethical aspects of pregnancy termination. I grew up in a country where termination of pregnancy was used as a means of birth control: in Poland, in its ostensibly Catholic society, it was accepted that obstetricians routinely provided abortions in their private offices. It was a fact of life and not a moral dilemma, but now that I was a geneticist offering prenatal diagnosis the potential fallout of my counselling was not lost on me. Babies were not born because of a diagnosis I had made, based on fuzzy grey ultrasound images, or on chromosomal analysis, or after consultation with other specialists. Because of the information I provided, some of these lives ended before they had even begun. I did not cause these abnormalities to happen, nature did. But what if I had been wrong? What if I misinterpreted an ultrasound image or a chromosome result? I had counselled so many pregnant women and so many of them chose to stop their pregnancies – had I, as this woman suggested, turned into a baby killer?

Once, I counselled a woman about an abnormal chromosome result after an amniocentesis – a finding called mixed polyploidy. The woman had undergone a routine amniocentesis because of her age, thirty-seven, but there were no signs on the ultrasound that the baby had a genetic condition. I had never heard about mixed polyploidy before, but Keith, our new cytogenetics scientist, handed me several articles that supported his interpretation. According to the papers, children with this chromosomal anomaly had a significant intellectual disability yet no birth defects and minimal dysmorphic features. Just like the baby in this woman's ultrasound.

It was the couple's first pregnancy and they were Roman Catholic. In spite of this, after I had explained the findings and what sort of future they could expect for their baby, they decided to stop the pregnancy. They met the obstetrician who would perform the procedure; they spoke with the social worker.

Two days later, on the morning of the scheduled termination, the chief technologist from the chromosome lab knocked on the door to my office. She wanted to talk about the fetus with polyploidy.

"The termination's today," I told her.

"That result isn't right," she said, her voice shaky. She straightened a stack of photocopied articles, tapping it against the surface of my desk. "You need to talk to them."

The abnormal result in the baby was, in fact, an artefact of growing the fetal cells in a laboratory culture, she told me. She had observed it many times before and the previous laboratory director had never reported those findings as abnormal. It was a known side effect of growing human cells in a petri dish. She showed me the articles that confirmed her interpretation. It was different if polyploidy was found in the blood sample from an older child – *then* it was associated with intellectual disability. Keith had shown me the papers on older children only.

"I tried to explain this to him but he wouldn't listen," the tech said.

That poor pregnant woman and her husband. I had put them through hell and now I had to find a way to take it all back, to undo it somehow. There was nobody I could ask for help. I had to face them myself and take back all that I had said.

I don't know how I did it, but I did do it.

The mother thanked me in the end, but I do not know if she or her husband ever trusted a medical professional after that.

☞

Clinical genetics made up the other half of my medical practice, and metabolics – the reason I went into genetics – the third. Yes, it somehow always happens that physicians' professional hours add up to more than two halves. I consulted on patients on the wards, in the neonatal intensive care unit and in my clinic. But when you combined the counsellors' supreme confidence with my non-existent confidence (I did not get a job at SickKids) and added to it my issues with self-worth (I did not get a job at SickKids) and the need to establish myself, you got quite the volatile mixture; fortunately, there were no explosions. At least no major ones.

I felt alone and isolated, with no mentors to guide or advise me, banished from the mecca of genetic research. Worse, I had no peers with whom to discuss cases, to learn from, to commiserate. Young and scared, I thought at first that I had to establish the pecking order with the genetic counsellors, prove myself worthy of being listened to, yet I had no idea how to do it. But as soon as I realized that the counsellors knew more than I did about genetic tests and counselling, I was wise enough to shut up and listen.

And then one February morning, two years after I started working at McMaster, the window brightly lit with sun bouncing off the fresh snow, I walked into my office to find a sheet of paper taped to my computer monitor; on it, a star jaggedly drawn in ballpoint pen. Susan, the genetic counsellor, stuck her head in after me and said that I had been a star. I had diagnosed correctly a rare – even by genetic standards – condition based on a photograph a pediatrician had shown me in passing, and the laboratory had just confirmed it. Susan was never stingy with praise – I just hadn't deserved it that often at the beginning.

In my clinical genetics practice, I revelled in intellectual challenges, in the feeling of accomplishment when all the pieces fit. I got a thrill when, during an autopsy of a baby with severe anomalies, I had asked if the baby had a cleft in his larynx. The pathologist had stared at me, impressed – yes, one of the walls of the baby's voice box was cleaved, cinching the diagnosis: Pallister-Hall syndrome. And when I told a grumpy, sceptical neurology professor what a girl's brain MRI would show based on her photograph, he came back a day later duly impressed because, indeed, the brain appeared abnormally smooth.

Sometimes, I diagnosed a condition on the spot, in an augenblick – a flash of recognition – or after a rapid rundown of the differential diagnosis tree. More often, however, I needed the help of computer databases, textbooks and genetics atlases. What a rush when the tests later confirmed my clinical diagnosis. I lived for that validation. Jimm even called me "House" for a while, after the television program of the same name. Dr. House specialized in diagnosing the rarest and strangest diseases. Although the moniker made me cringe – my bedside manner was humane, not absurd like his – I did recognize that Jimm was complimenting my cerebral abilities and not commenting on my personality.

My brain did not stop naming syndromes when I stepped outside the hospital. It diagnosed Jack's daycare worker, who had the webbed neck and hooded eyelids of Noonan syndrome. It recognized the four-foot-ten sales clerk at a duty-free shop at Amsterdam's Schiphol Airport as having hypochondroplasia, a not-uncommon form of dwarfism. The usher at Vicenza's famed theatre had the windswept knees of pseudoachondroplasia; the boy sitting in a wheelchair at the Blue Jays' game, the twisted limbs of arthrogryposis. Of course, I never ran after anybody in the mall to share my diagnoses; it was just a brain game. But I did say something to the father of a newborn I examined in the NICU one winter, after debating with myself for several minutes whether I should, whether I had the right. While examining his daughter, I had recognized in him the coarsened facial features of acromegaly, a potentially lethal but treatable endocrine condition. I had hesitated because he was not my patient, but in the end, I decided that I could ask him whether he had ever seen a hormone specialist. When he said no, I explained to him what I saw and made an urgent referral to an internist. A few months later, he sent me a long, grateful letter after a neurosurgeon removed a tumour from his pituitary gland, saving his sight.

I have always had a need to be the best and to be recognized as such. But wanting to be praised had been a moving target. During my childhood, my mother and various teachers all had different expectations of me, and I missed the mark most of the time. My conduct in school, for which we were marked, was my Achilles' heel. I was a tomboy; I was unruly, talked out of turn, couldn't sit still. It might have been because I was bored – my behaviours improved somewhat when I was allowed to skip grade four. My mother berated me every time I brought home a note from the teacher or she had to make the trip to school to "discuss me." I kept trying to please her, and finally, in grade five, arrived at what I thought was a foolproof method of securing her acceptance: perfect marks. I had no other talents; I was a hopeless klutz in sports and had a wooden ear for the piano (my mother had insisted on lessons). In Canada, my isolation and the desire to get into medical school only abetted my perfectionist tendencies, as did medical school itself and my perceived failures there. And since I was now too old to be wishing for approval from my mother, I shifted that need to my colleagues.

The general attitude among other specialists is that geneticists spend a lot of time doing nothing. Only a physician who has experienced genetic counselling firsthand understands why it takes an hour to explain a genetic condition and its inheritance to a patient. No other consultants – except psychiatrists – spend that much time with a patient. To some, this talking is not real medicine.

In the weeks leading up to Christmas, my medical and surgical colleagues would parade through the hospital corridors laden with bottles of wine and boxes of chocolate wrapped in festive red-and-green or white-and-silver paper. I have never received a Christmas gift from a patient. It used to bother me – for most of December, my colleague's office is a cornucopia of chocolate boxes, wine bottles, jars of candy. But he follows patients with metabolic disorders and actually "does something" for them. It has taken many years for me to realize that my pediatric colleagues do respect me, and that neonatologists and the NICU nurses appreciate the caring and warm (or so they say) way that I counsel parents and deliver to them terrible diagnoses. But this realization was a long time in coming.

Early in my clinical career, I followed Brendan, a boy with Beckwith-Wiedemann syndrome. I had initially been consulted on his mother's pregnancy because the prenatal ultrasound detected an omphalocele – a large opening in the middle of the abdomen that allows the intestines and sometimes the liver to protrude outside the body, covered only by a membrane – and an enlarged tongue. After his birth, genetic testing confirmed my clinical diagnosis. Children with this syndrome have an increased risk of developing tumours of the kidney and liver, and, until the age of seven, require ultrasound scans of their abdomen and blood work every three months in order to monitor for nascent malignancy. Brendan's surveillance continued uneventfully for four years, until one day he just did not look right. With dark circles under his eyes, he slumped on the chair in my clinic room, listless, holding his mother's hand. He was pale, his face drawn.

"He's been droopy like that for about three weeks," his mother said. "His pediatrician said it was anemia and prescribed iron."

My gut was telling me it was something else. I always listen to my gut – the two times that I ignored it, I found out later that it had been right. Since then, a red light flashes for me whenever my brain tells me to ignore my gut. Gut says, Something's wrong; brain says, Eh, nothing to worry about; I say, Check it out, fast. Never fails.

No need for the internal struggle that time: Brendan was sick. He had a low-grade fever and his pulse fluttered like a bird's.

"I think that he's lost some weight, too," his mother said.

I ordered an urgent ultrasound of his abdomen, thinking I would find a tumour in his belly. It showed that the lymph nodes along Brendan's aorta were big and boggy-looking – the radiologist wondered about leukemia or lymphoma. But from his previous sonograms, I had known that Brendan had a cyst in his left kidney. I ordered an urgent biopsy of the cyst. The syringe pulled back yellow, bloody pus – bacteria had seeded into the cyst, a not-uncommon complication. Brendan's body was managing to keep it under control but at the expense of his iron levels, fevers and fatigue. The lymph nodes were swollen because they were fighting off the infection – it was not a lymphoma, thank goodness. I admitted Brendan to the hospital, and after two weeks of intravenous antibiotics, the infection cleared and a surgeon resected the cyst.

A few weeks later, I ran into Brendan and his mother at the hospital entrance. Brendan was carrying a bunch of flowers and a festively wrapped box. His mother greeted me in passing and they proceeded to the surgeon's office.

I hope the surgeon enjoyed the chocolates.

☞

At McMaster, I continued to photograph my patients but this time with a significant difference. The misgivings I had experienced about the ethics of clinical photography during my fellowship found a counterpart in a question Susan had asked the first time I was setting up to shoot a photo of a patient. The patient had Aarskog syndrome, with widely spaced eyes, a widow's peak and short stature, as well as webbed fingers.

"You're going to get a consent, aren't you?" she more stated than asked. And she handed me a form.

Until that moment, I had never heard of a consent form for taking clinical photographs. No parent or patient signed one at SickKids. They implied consent by their actions as they picked up the yellow requisition and rode the elevator to the photography studio. At McMaster Children's Hospital, however, the consent form was printed on the back of the photograph requisition itself. It had to be signed by a parent or guardian before the audiovisual department would photograph the patient. Checkboxes stipulated whether the photos were for "clinical treatment only," "research purposes including publication" or "publicity purposes of the hospital."

Requesting a signature on the consent form removed the discomfort I had experienced but never admitted to at SickKids. I had never questioned the practice of photographing patients, but the moment the counsellor queried me, I realized that the unease had been there all along. One could want to have a great teaching slide collection, one could want to document clinical features and to publish cases, yet feel uneasy about it at the same time.

Most parents signed the form without much thought. Many said that they didn't need the consent, that they trusted me. But for some, it offered an opportunity to refuse. At first, I thought that the consent itself acted as a deterrent – that the parents felt uncomfortable with the legality, the officialness of the signature, not with the photos themselves. In those difficult-to-diagnose cases, a refusal annoyed me – didn't they realize how important a diagnosis was? How it would help their child? At first, I assumed that they worried that the photo would be published without their knowledge.

"It's for documentation only." I would point to the box that I had ticked off.

"No, it's okay," they would answer in the positive-negative manner of steadfast refusal, and it would dawn on me that they simply did not want to have the photo taken and nothing I said would change their mind. I quickly learned not to insist.

In documenting patients' features, I embraced digital photography as soon as it became semi-affordable. In 1997, my department provided funds to buy a silver Olympus, one of the first digital cameras on the market. It resembled a toucan with a lens screwed at the end of its silver beak. Macro step lenses allowed me to shoot magnified photos of fetuses after termination of pregnancy so that their minuscule features would be visible. With digital photography, there was no need for film processing and printing, no need to worry about unauthorized access during the developing process. After shooting, I downloaded the images onto the firewalled hospital server. Since then, I have progressed from the clunky Olympus through a series of automated Nikons and SLRs to my iPhone, each much more optically and technologically advanced than my silver toucan. And since taking photographs with a phone may appear cavalier and unprofessional, I assure parents that the phone is password-protected as well, and that the images are erased the moment I download them onto the firewalled hard drive: "The photographs are part of the confidential medical records and protected by the same privacy policies."

No more three-ring binders with clear pockets for slides, no more affixing labels by hand, no more hand-writing labels. Stored in my office, I have ten CDs, one for each year, with photographs burned onto them from the time when burning CDs was the technology *du jour*. The most recent ones live on an external hard drive.

Within two or three years, I stopped taking photographs of known conditions – I had amassed a sufficient collection for teaching residents and fellows. But I did use the slides that I had collected until then to teach the pediatric residents that rotated through the genetics service. I also inaugurated a series of dysmorphology rounds, which were very popular and which, together with my teaching during the rotations, garnered me the McMaster Pediatric Residency Teaching Award in 1998.

I still photographed rare findings, rare conditions and patients I couldn't diagnose so that I could consult with other geneticists. But again, after reviewing more than a hundred cases at sessions at genetics conferences devoted to diagnostic unknowns or via encrypted emails with colleagues, I realized that if I couldn't diagnose a patient, others probably would not be able to, either. The patient either had a novel condition, worthy of publication, or the condition was just too rare or too non-specific to be recognized even by an experienced clinical geneticist.

Photos of patients I cannot diagnose give me a chance to review their features, to reconsider details, to revise my thinking. Sometimes, when I examine the photographs in my office, I notice a feature – the appearance of the nose in profile, the shape of the eyes and eyebrows – I might have missed during the physical examination in the clinic. The stillness of the photo highlights subtle features invisible when a child wiggles in their mother's lap or scurries around the examination room. I return to the photos time and time again, hoping that a key piece of the puzzle will fall into place, that I might find the right clue that will lead me to order a test that will deliver a diagnosis.

For several years now, I have been wondering what to do with the seven three-ring binders of patients' slides that have begun to gather dust on a shelf in my office. I'd used them to teach residents how to recognize dysmorphic features – I would show them a photograph and ask whether the person in the photo had dysmorphic features. Only after the residents committed themselves to an answer would I review the photograph in detail and point out which of the patient's features made the resident notice the difference. Upward-slanting palpebral fissures – the eyes slant upwards.

Anteverted nares – a turned-up nose with the nostrils pointing forward instead of down. Through this photographic tutelage, the students also learned the vocabulary to describe different features.

But photographs are no longer physical objects; they are billions and trillions of ones and zeros encoding each image, its colour, its tragedy, on camera storage cards, on laptops and computers, and online. The physical has become ethereal, and the images of patients' bodies have become electronic ghosts that will live on forever. Today, every syndrome ever described can be found online within microseconds of a mouse click, illustrated with photos often technically better than those in my collection. Many photos of children with syndromes are posted by their parents in online parents' groups. Others are published in medical journals; some are of patients who I know. Through my university library's subscriptions, at my desktop computer, I have access to a vast collection of medical journals and countless photographs. If I cannot find a good illustration of a particular clinical feature in my files, I am certain to locate one by typing its name into Google. These days, a new geneticist can amass an entire teaching collection without examining a single patient. My slide collection, once so obsessively curated, has become obsolete and is gathering dust on the shelf in my office.

What should I do with all those slides? I cannot use them for teaching anymore – there is only one slide projector available in our hospital's audiovisual department, and when I switch it on it sounds like a dilapidated tractor struggling up a steep hill. Remember those fans that kept the projector bulb from overheating? That sound. I cannot use the photos for an art project honouring the patients or publish them in a commemorative album – a suggestion from a patients' rights advocate – since I have never obtained consent for such use. I will have to decide what to do with those photos before I retire and vacate my office. But I am not ready to let go of them yet. Each is a window into a human story, an illustration of a single facet of the experience of being human.

☞

When I arrived at McMaster, the metabolic diseases practice there oper-ated completely differently from the one at SickKids. There were no ded-icated fellows or residents on the service, so all questions on hospitalized patients were directed to the attending physician, including requests for Tylenol at two in the morning. One sick two-month-old with an organic acidemia – a metabolic disorder causing a buildup of acids in the body's fluids – could keep me on the ward or in the ICU all weekend. Soon, the sheer volume of clinical work began to tarnish the shine of figuring out obscure biochemical pathways. But I persevered – it was what I had always wanted to do.

At least until Clara arrived from Kitchener with yet another crisis.

She was an eleven-year-old girl with a urea cycle disorder in which a liver enzyme that converts ammonia, a toxic by-product of protein breakdown, into the water-soluble urea eliminated in the urine, is not functioning. Don Whelan had diagnosed her when she was just three days old. Clara had weathered many hospital admissions, both at McMaster and at the local hospital in Kitchener-Waterloo, yet she never lost her sense of humour. Because patients with elevated blood ammonia could become confused and disoriented as the first sign of worsening, during the first twenty-four hours the nurses woke her up her every two hours. One way to assess a patient's wherewithal is to ask for their name and whether they know the date and where they are.

This time Clara seemed fine except for vomiting – another sign of elevated ammonia. When children with urea cycle disorder do not eat, their bodies break down their own muscle proteins for calories and ammonia rises even higher, which makes them sicker and even less able to keep anything down – a vicious circle. The only way to break through this pattern is to admit the patient to the hospital, where sugars and lipids and ammonia-lowering drugs can be given intravenously without relying on the sick gut.

I examined Clara around 5:00 p.m. She was a bit groggy, but her afternoon blood ammonia measured lower than at admission and she had not vomited the apple juice her mom had given her an hour earlier. I joked with Clara and chatted with her mom, reviewed the medication and intravenous orders with the nurses and the resident on call, then went home.

That evening, Jimm and I managed to get Jack to sleep shortly after eight – a miracle – and then settled in for an evening of reading and catching up on dictating patients' charts. We didn't have a nanny because Jimm vetoed the idea. He preferred to have Jack in daycare where we were held accountable to how late we would be picking him up. Every morning, Jimm dropped Jack off at a daycare near his hospital and picked him in the late afternoon. But when Jack wasn't well, I would be the one to receive the phone call, even though my hospital was halfway across the city. We hadn't been able to find a babysitter, and when one was available it was on weekends when we had to go to work. We had no help from anybody, so by the time evenings arrived, all of us – except Jack, that is – were exhausted. But there was no rest for the weary – Jack still wasn't sleeping through the night.

That night, I phoned the ward around 11:00 p.m., just before Jimm and I switched off the lights. Clara was sleeping. Jack woke up after midnight and it took him his usual forty minutes to fall back asleep. Ever since he was an infant, he would not settle easily after nighttime feedings; Jimm or I had to pace with him until he fell asleep in our arms and then repeat the whole process three hours later. For an absurd period of about two months, sitting on a running clothes dryer was the only thing we could find that would soothe him – the vibrations transmitted through our bodies lulled him. But he would jerk awake the moment we slid off the dryer. And each morning, he woke up at 6:00 a.m. on the dot. By the time Clara was admitted to McMaster, Jimm and I had not had a good night's sleep for fourteen months.

My pager beeped around 3:00 a.m. Lucy, the pediatric resident on call for Clara's ward, sounded worried and upset.

"Clara's agitated, her mother can't settle her," Lucy said. In the background, I heard Clara's yells, but they barely registered in my muddled consciousness. I slumped against the kitchen counter, where I had staggered so as not to wake Jimm, the cabinets above me swimming in and out of focus. I could not keep my eyes open no matter how hard I rubbed them or how many times I blinked. "Sleep, must go to sleep," repeated in my head on a loop. I can't think, I can't take this, what am I supposed to do, I can't think. If I could only lie down, be horizontal, head on a pillow, what? Lucy said something I didn't catch.

"I'm worried about her IV access." If Clara lost her intravenous line, we couldn't treat her.

"What's her intake?" I asked, but again I did not follow the numbers Lucy recited. "And her midnight ammonia?" The number Lucy gave me was fine, only a unit or two higher than that afternoon's value.

My mind reeled. I need to sleep or I won't function tomorrow, I have a full clinic in the morning. What?

"Ativan?" I said. "Yes, give her half a dose and see if it helps."

I have no recollection as to how I got back upstairs and into bed.

Five hours later, I arrived on the ward before morning rounds. Clara was still asleep, her mother standing by her bed.

"I can't wake her," Clara's mother said.

Clara was comatose. She did not respond when I rubbed her breast-bone or pinched her toes. Her ammonia level, the lab notified us a half-hour later, had risen to three times normal. I arranged for an immediate transfer to the ICU for dialysis to clear the blood of ammonia, but it was too late: her brain had swollen and filled her skull to capacity. Within two hours, she needed a respirator to breathe for her because the swollen brain tissues had squeezed out through the opening in the bottom of her skull like tooth-paste out of a tube and had crushed the breathing centre in her brainstem. Clara never regained consciousness, and two days later the ICU physicians declared her brain-dead. Her parents now had to make the worst decision in the world: to stop their daughter's life support.

The ICU physician was preparing to switch off the respirator. Silence filled the cubicle where Clara lay. I lingered by the door, not wanting to breach the tight wreath of relatives around Clara's bed, but her father noticed me, let go of his wife's hand and extended his arm toward me. They pulled me closer, and between them I watched as Clara's chest rose for the last time and her heartbeat slowed to nothing. They wanted me there, even though I felt I did not deserve it. I thought that I had failed Clara. I should have gone into the hospital that night, come away from my sleep and from my son. I should have done something more, something sooner, something better.

Exhausted and wrung out like a dirty dishtowel, I called Jimm to pick me up. On the way home, we passed Clara's parents walking alone, hand in hand, toward Ronald McDonald House where they were staying. My heart broke at the sight of their clasped hands. They were good, kind people who didn't deserve what had happened. Neither did their daughter.

Clara's funeral was held in Kitchener four days later. Banners and posters of photos decked the walls of the funeral parlour. The Clara I had never known smiled from all of them. Her parents hugged me, hugged Don and thanked us for the wonderful care that Clara had always received at McMaster.

I felt like a complete fraud, and worse, an incompetent.

By the time I was pregnant with my second son the following year, Don Whelan had retired and Dr. Murray Potter, who would take over the metabolics service, was still completing his training at BC Children's Hospital in Vancouver. I was the only physician trained in the two subspecialties but no way could I – or anybody else, for that matter – be physically capable of covering both services alone, even for a short period of time. I requested that the care of the metabolic patients be temporarily transferred to SickKids or to London Children's Hospital. "I have a small son at home and another on the way," I told the hospital administration. "I can't do metabolics and genetics and prenatal."

The administration agreed. For five months, until Murray became a staff physician in July 2002, our patients with metabolic diseases travelled to SickKids for emergencies and routine care. And when he started, I chose not to share the metabolic call with him – I couldn't face another Clara.

Until now, I never told anybody the real reason I quit metabolic genetics, my dream specialty.

8

A university appointment comes with many demands. Sometimes too many. Apart from doing what a geneticist does in a community hospital – consulting and caring for patients on the wards and in clinics, and supervising genetic counsellors – an academic physician also has a responsibility to teach medical students and pediatric residents, and to advance the knowledge of human disease by conducting research and publishing findings. Ever since medical school, I had known that I wanted to do all those things.

Jimm also had academic aspirations. After two more years as a clinical scholar, he was finally offered a position as a full-time physician on a university faculty, where he was ideally placed to climb the academic ladder. Within a few years, he was conducting multi-million-dollar clinical research studies; was published in *The New England Journal of Medicine*, the highest-impact internal medicine journal in the world; and became the world-recognized expert on blood clots that he is. By now, having published almost four hundred peer-reviewed medical articles, he travels around the world delivering lectures at conferences and meetings, holds a research chair in thromboembolic disease at McMaster University and is the president of Thrombosis Canada, a national medical organization dedicated to blood clot prevention, treatment and education, among many other accomplishments. We have always shared child care and household duties equally and concentrated our attention on work and raising our sons. For fun, Jimm plays cello in a community orchestra and I read voraciously; we have no social life to speak of.

During my genetics fellowship, I published four case reports of rare or newly discovered genetic conditions, but case reports were not enough to sustain a university research career. Once at McMaster, I fretted about academic productivity, the dreaded "publish or perish" axiom, and about my academic advancement. The academic rank of an assistant professor, the rank that I received at McMaster University, is granted to any physician with a pulse who is hired at an academic hospital. I wanted to be better than that – I wanted a promotion to associate professor, to show my academic mettle. But since I had no research ideas or opportunities, I continued to publish case reports, considered the lowest rung in the hierarchy of scientific papers, and lost sleep over the prospects for my academic future.

Until a pediatrician requested a consultation on a newborn girl with a cleft palate.

☞

Aleesha was born by C-section in the week leading to Christmas 1998. From the moment she was born, she spluttered and choked while feeding and food came out of her nose. She was two days old when the nurses discovered a hole in her hard palate. It is a paradox of embryology that when associated with a cleft lip, cleft palate is seldom caused by an underlying genetic condition, even though it appears much, much worse. Such a defect right in the middle of a newborn face leaves the child with the curled red buds of the split upper lip and the shell-like pink walls of the exposed nasal cavity. But in a cleft palate *without* a cleft lip, serious genetic syndromes lurk, many associated with intellectual disability, hidden out of sight just like the cleft palate itself.

"Do you know why I'm here?" I asked Lore, Aleesha's mother.

She eyed me suspiciously. My visits are seldom welcome, especially in the newborn nursery. No new mother wants to consider that there may be something genetically wrong with her just-born baby.

"She has a cleft palate," she said, so quietly I barely heard her.

"Whenever a baby is born with a birth difference a geneticist is asked to assess the baby. It's routine." I did not want to scare her any more than she already was.

Aleesha weighed 1,800 grams – about two and a half pounds, tiny for a full-term baby. Her minuscule jaw and small, recessed chin had caused the cleft palate. As the mouth cavity develops, the two shelves of the palate grow from the sides and knit together in the middle. In an under-grown, underdeveloped jaw, the tongue bunches up in the middle of the mouth and prevents the palate from closing, a condition called Robin sequence. Aleesha had Robin sequence. Even in the penumbra of the patient's room, with dim light slanting from above Lore's headboard, I noticed that Aleesha also had a short nose with nostrils that faced forward, droopy eyelids and ears that sat low on her skull. Her forehead was narrow and her head appeared small. To the untrained eye, she looked adorable. And I told Lore that.

But I recognized the syndrome, even though I had never examined a patient with it. Only three years earlier, the discovery of the biochemical defect underlying Smith-Lemli-Opitz syndrome (named after the three physicians who first described it in 1964, the year I was born) turned the entire field of dysmorphology on its head. It was the first ever condition caused by an enzyme deficiency that resulted in abnormal facial features and birth defects. And its underlying defect – a blockage in the last step of cholesterol production in the body – put the entire field of cholesterol research on *its* head, too, because it turned out that rather than being the all-time dietary bad guy, cholesterol was essential to the normal development of the human embryo, especially its brain. At the time, I had devoured all the papers on the subject; many of them had photographs of babies with the exact features that I was now seeing in the newborn before me.

To be sure, I needed to examine her.

I reached for Aleesha. "May I?" I asked.

Lore glanced at the baby sleeping peacefully in her arms like she did not want to let me touch her. What goes through the mind of a mother that surrenders her newborn to an examination that might find something wrong? I cannot imagine. Did she suspect that this was the last moment of her so-called normal life?

She opened her arms, her unwillingness almost palpable.

I lay Aleesha in her bassinet. Wrapped tightly in a white receiving blanket speckled with yellow flowers, she resembled a swaddled little tamale.

I eased out her tiny hand – yes, she had the stubby thumb with underdeveloped muscles at its base. I unwrapped her, undressed her – not a whimper. I examined every inch of her, even though I only needed to see her feet – her second and third toes started as one and then branched into two ends topped with tiny pearly nails. This was the telltale sign: Aleesha had Smith-Lemli-Opitz syndrome.

I rewrapped her and handed her back to Lore, who hugged her to her chest.

"Aleesha has some findings that I need to check out," I said.

"What does she have?" Lore was having none of my prevarication.

"It's called Smith-Lemli-Opitz syndrome, after the three doctors who discovered it. There's a blood test that will tell us for sure. It'll be a week or so before we'll have it back."

Lore glared at me. "How can you be so sure?" She sounded angry.

"I'm not," I lied. "That's why we need to do the test." I wanted to give Lore time to get used to the idea.

At the nurses' station, I ordered a test for 7DHC, the abnormal metabolite I expected to find in Aleesha's blood. High levels of 7DHC in Aleesha's blood would confirm the diagnosis.

I also ordered a karyotype, a chromosomal study – some boys with a severe form of Smith-Lemli-Opitz syndrome have underdeveloped genitalia and could appear as girls in spite of having male chromosomes. I sincerely hoped that this was not a case – telling a parent that a baby girl is actually a baby boy or vice versa is one of the hardest things a geneticist has to do.

Aleesha's chromosomes were female, but she did have Smith-Lemli-Opitz syndrome. I met with Lore and Paul, Aleesha's father, the following week. As I explained the genetics and the biochemistry of their daughter's condition, Lore's lips were drawn in a tight line. Did she hate me now? When I offered a second opinion from a colleague or from another genetics centre, she shook her head. I think she didn't want to hear it again.

"No," she said, not meeting my eye. "I believe you."

Smith-Lemli-Opitz syndrome had entered my consciousness while at the American Society of Human Genetics meeting in Montreal in 1995, which also happened to be the first society meeting I attended.

Five thousand-plus researchers, physicians and counsellors milled around the four floors of the Palais des congrès de Montréal. Thousands of scientific posters describing the most recent findings and observations and research hung in the massive, brightly lit exhibit halls, their walls removed to make one huge hall larger than an airport hangar. Over the four days, more than two hundred lectures ran in concurrent sessions – I wished I could have cloned myself. I tried to attend as many as I could, to read and discuss as many posters in clinical and metabolic genetics as possible, only to collapse, brain full, at night in my hotel room, struggling to process and retain what I had seen and heard. The evening sessions were still running, scheduled until 10:00 p.m. I had never attended a lecture as large as the plenary sessions or the presidential address, the attending members seated in a darkened room the size of a football field, three Jumbotrons projecting images of the speakers. I wanted to know it all, yet all too soon I realized it was futile – my brain filled to capacity within the first day.

And then I heard about Smith-Lemli-Opitz syndrome.

"Imagine," said Debbie, a SickKids genetics fellow who was also in attendance, "a biochemical defect that causes a malformation syndrome."

"What?" I pricked my ears. This was my bailiwick – I was the only one of the four fellows who'd dedicated a whole year of study to biochemical genetics. What Debbie said made no sense: enzyme deficiencies did not cause birth defects; mutation in genes for structural proteins did. Until then, biochemistry and dysmorphology did not overlap.

"Smith-Lemli-Opitz syndrome," Debbie said. "Characteristic facial features, multiple birth defects, intellectual disability. Known for years and now discovered to be caused by a defect in the synthesis of cholesterol."

"How?" I asked.

"That's it – nobody knows. And it could be treatable, like the other biochemical disorders." I knew that birth defects could not be undone – once organs formed along the wrong blueprints, they were set in stone. But maybe an intellectual disability could be prevented? Or even – reversed? Cured? I sat there, amazed and awed by the possible implications.

The following month, back in Toronto, Debbie and her supervisor diagnosed Smith-Lemli-Opitz syndrome in an eighteen-year-old man; the biochemical test confirmed it. Debbie wrote up a research protocol and presented it to the SickKids Ethics Board for approval. I wished I had seen that patient. I wished I had a research project on the disease of the moment, but it was Debbie who had picked up his chart from the pile that morning. Luck is just as important as training or brains in making a research career.

☞

It so happened that five weeks before I examined Aleesha, Don Whelan had diagnosed Smith-Lemli-Opitz syndrome in two brothers, eighteen-month-old Mitchell and two-and-a-half-year-old Daniel. Three children with the condition that absolutely fascinated me – I would have to be crazy not to run with it.

Don, nearing retirement, agreed to transfer the brothers to my care. Nobody questioned my suitability or my motivation in trying to become an expert in Smith-Lemli-Opitz syndrome like I'm sure would have happened with the establishment at SickKids. At McMaster, if I wanted to, I could do the extra work as long as the care of other patients did not suffer. I didn't have to jump through administrative hoops at departmental and hospital levels; I didn't have to compete with anybody. I reread three years' worth of papers in lipid and cholesterol research, and all the publications on Smith-Lemli-Opitz syndrome before and since the discovery of the biochemical defect. Cholesterol therapy had already been tested in clinical trials in the United States, so I started Aleesha, Daniel and Mitchell on dietary cholesterol supplements. The McMaster pharmacist prepared the suspension based on a formula used by Dr. Richard Kelley at the Kennedy Krieger Institute in Baltimore. Nobody had an ego, nobody put up roadblocks, and Richard shared his cholesterol formula with me freely.

In June 1999, I travelled to Salt Lake City to attend the Smith-Lemli-Opitz Foundation meeting where families of children with Smith-Lemli-Opitz syndrome mingled with geneticists and researchers. Except for Gail, Mitchell and Daniel's mother, I was the only Canadian there.

Nothing compares to seeing two dozen or so people with a supposedly once-in-a-lifetime condition crowded into a single room. Most physicians will never meet a single person with Smith-Lemli-Opitz syndrome and there I sat, perched on a sofa in Salt Lake City University Park Marriott's five-storey lobby overrun by them. Babies in car seats, stomach pumps whirring quietly beside them; older children in wheelchairs. The ones able to walk were loping and lurching - children with Smith-Lemli-Opitz syndrome have a characteristic gait: hunched, their arms flexed and head perched forward on their necks, they teeter as if about to fall. And then they take a step. Then another. One afternoon, I snuck into the playroom where the infants and children there displayed all of the unusual behaviours of Smith-Lemli-Opitz syndrome: inconsolable crying, screaming, throwing themselves backward against walls, autistic-like twirling and hand flapping. Kids with Smith-Lemli-Opitz syndrome scream all night, they bite their own arms and hands, but they never hurt anyone other than themselves. Lore and Gail lived with that every day and night. I have no idea how they managed it.

At that meeting, I also met Dr. John Opitz himself, one of the fathers of North American genetics. An immigrant from Germany, he has made his home in the United States for fifty years. He was a legend among clinical geneticists, at least a half-dozen syndromes bore his name, either alone or paired with those of other genetics giants. On Saturday morning, the geneticists attending the conference and local pediatricians of various specialities consulted on patients in the hospital clinics. He and I saw a young man who'd come to the conference with the diagnosis of Smith-Lemli-Opitz syndrome but clearly didn't have it.

"What do you think he has?" John asked me, clearly in his teacher role.

"FG syndrome," I said. Also known as Opitz-Kaveggia syndrome, it was another of the syndromes he had described. But John didn't like eponymic names so I wisely avoided it.

He smiled. "I think so, too," he said.

☞

When three groups of scientists discovered the gene for Smith-Lemli-Opitz syndrome a year later, I photocopied the scientific reports and, articles in hand, barged into Dr. John Waye's office. John is the director of the McMaster Molecular Genetics laboratory and a world expert on the DNA diagnostics of thalassemias and sickle cell disease, genetic conditions that cause anemia. Our offices share a wall.

"How would you like to set up a diagnostic test for SLOS?" I asked.

"Okay," he said, and, after a beat, "What's a SLOS?"

That was it. At SickKids, I probably would have had to plead my case to seven and a half committees and prepare eleventeen detailed analyses on how the test would affect laboratory resources and personnel; at McMaster, I only needed to traipse down the hall and ask.

"I'll need positive controls," John said. "Get me those and we'll set it up."

Sure. Positive controls are blood samples from individuals in whom the genetic test has already been performed and validated. Every lab that tests biological specimens needs positive controls to ensure that their test is working. Where could I get those?

Help came from the place I would have least expected – Poland. In Warsaw, Professor Małgorzata Krajewska-Walasek, the head of the National Children's Health Institute genetics clinic, had recently published her experience with thirteen Polish patients, including their genetic results. Having never met the woman, I emailed the address listed in the journal's byline and asked whether she would be willing to share samples from her patients with us. She agreed. A month later, a small cardboard box wrapped in industrial grade plastic, affixed with an orange BIOHAZARD sticker and a wad of customs forms arrived at McMaster: samples of DNA from six confirmed Polish patients with SLOS. I carried the box to the molecular laboratory like it was platinum alloyed with gold and studded with diamonds. Within a month, the chief DNA technician, Barry Eng, developed and validated molecular genetic testing of Smith-Lemli-Opitz syndrome in our laboratory – the first time this had been done in Canada. We were ready.

☞

Within a year, buoyed by the success of establishing the DNA diagnostics at McMaster and buzzing from the Salt Lake City meeting, I developed two research ideas: a national surveillance for patients with Smith-Lemli-Opitz syndrome and a study of its facial features. The surveillance would determine how many children with Smith-Lemli-Opitz syndrome were born in Canada each year and how many were still alive – infants with the most severe form of the syndrome often lived only a few months if not weeks. The Canadian Paediatric Surveillance Program run by the Canadian Paediatric Society had been established expressly for the surveillance of very rare conditions such as SLOS. Every month, the society's members receive a form on which they check off whether they have treated any children with the conditions under study. In the '90s, it was by post; now the surveillance is run by email. Positive responses are returned to researchers for further study. At that time, in the late 1990s, the program cost eighteen thousand dollars a year for each disorder, and in order to obtain statistically meaningful results, I calculated that the surveillance for Smith-Lemli-Opitz syndrome had to continue for at least three years. I began to write a research grant proposal to fund it and to prepare a presentation for the McMaster University Research Ethics Board.

That fall, the 1999 annual meeting of the American Society of Human Genetics was held in San Francisco. I had submitted three abstracts for the meeting and taught myself to use PowerPoint to design posters. On top of seeing patients in clinic and consulting on prenatal cases and newborns in our NICU, I effortlessly flew through computer files, graphs and photographs; edited the text and figure labels; and ensured that, together with all the necessary references, my presentations fit onto the three-by-four-foot poster boards for display. On October 19, after four hours of sleep, I got up at 4:00 a.m. to catch the eight o'clock flight from Pearson International Airport. When the plane touched down in San Francisco, the grey concrete of the Oakland Bay Bridge shimmering in the late-morning sun, I was buzzing with energy. During the five-hour flight, I had read almost five hundred abstracts in clinical, prenatal and biochemical genetics without even once getting up from my seat. After checking into Le Méridien hotel, Marlene, with whom I shared a room, and I hit the city: we rode the famed trolley to the harbourfront, barked at the seals at Fisherman's Wharf (well, I did) and ate clam chowder in a sourdough bread bowl, Alcatraz shimmering in the sun as it flooded the bay. Afterward, I ran through the San Francisco MoMA and its store before the evening's opening reception.

Over three days at the Moscone Center, lectures, presentations and workshops blurred together with get-togethers and catching up with friends from around the world. Unlike the meeting the year before – when I felt unaccomplished and banished to Hamilton – I radiated confidence in my abilities and knowledge, and looked forward to my future accomplishments of which I was certain. If somebody had strummed me with a pick, I would have sung out like a well-tuned guitar. I talked about SLOS to anybody who'd listen, caught up with Denny Porter and Chris Wassif – the researchers from National Institutes of Health I had met at the Salt Lake City conference – and took pages and pages of notes in every lecture I attended.

The evening of the final gala, after which I was to board a 6:00 a.m. flight back to Toronto, I found myself in the hotel room of a recently divorced colleague, splayed out half-naked on the crisp sheets of his queen-size bed, drunk out of my skull. His room on the twenty-eighth floor of the just-opened W Hotel exuded über cool – its furniture had a New York vibe, its bathroom a vaguely European one. Even though I spent most of the night kneeling on its chic black-and-white-tiled bathroom floor vomiting into the toilet, and even though I kept my underwear on, for the first time since meeting Jimm I spent a night with another man. By 5:00 a.m., I had sobered up enough to be escorted back to my own hotel, where I threw my clothes into a suitcase, grabbed my thick file of notes from the desk and ran to catch a cab to the airport. I slept my drunkenness off on the flight back to Toronto, my head propped on the tray in front of me. Luckily, I had a window seat.

Once back home, I ran with my projects with equal intensity. To enrol Canadian geneticists who were not members of the Canadian Paediatric Society into the surveillance program, I called every last one – from

St. John's to Victoria – to cajole them into agreeing to participate. I left messages with their offices, paged them, called again. I pulled into parking lots on the way home from daycare, Jack strapped in his car seat, to answer pages. Honey dripped off my tongue once I had a colleague on the line, and eventually everybody signed up to receive the monthly mailings. In the evenings, I typed notes from my conference scribbles. A week after returning from San Francisco, I delivered a lecture in the Sheraton Fallsview Hotel in Niagara – without relying on notes – on the behavioural features of Smith-Lemli-Opitz syndrome at the fully packed annual conference of the National Association for the Dually Diagnosed. I invited myself into friends' homes at ten o'clock at night and kept them talking 'til well past midnight. I bummed cigarettes off those who smoked.

Soon, I had lost so much weight I could pull off my jeans fully zipped and buttoned. Sex with Jimm blew my mind, but whenever he asked me to take care of Jack or make dinner or clean up the house, I would sprout fangs and talons, and horns would spring from my head. I had better things to do than look after a child and a household. I wrote and submitted papers based on the posters I had presented in San Francisco. I stayed up nights and knit an Aran scarf cabled with the DNA double helix.

After a month of this wild roller-coaster ride, Jimm demanded I call Dr. Whitfield, my old psychiatrist in Toronto. He threatened to take Jack and move out if I didn't. To shut up his incessant harping, I made an appointment. On the way to Dr. Whitfield's office, I stopped at Tiffany's on Bloor Street in Toronto to shop for Christmas presents, buying Jimm a watch and my parents an Elsa Peretti crystal bowl – stretching our budget and Visa credit. I took the time to inspect the Bloor Street shop windows and enjoy the Christmas lights. I arrived only twenty-five minutes late for my appointment.

Dr. Whitfield's steady gaze followed me as I paced behind the sofa on which I used to sit during my years of therapy. Words poured out of me, unstoppable: I did not know why Jimm wanted me to see her, I was fine; I loved writing papers, publishing articles, applying for research grants; I was on the cusp of a major professional and research breakthrough; I did not need to be here; I had to go back to my office in Hamilton to tend to my patients who needed me; this was a complete waste of time.

She did not agree: less than forty-eight hours later, I had an appointment with Dr. Lawrence Martin, the head of the Mood Disorders Clinic at McMaster. I had to ask Don Whelan to see my clinic patients that morning – a stupid and unnecessary inconvenience for us both, I believed. During his consultation, Dr. Martin didn't know whether I was experiencing a midlife crisis – I was turning thirty-five in less than a month, after all – or exhibiting symptoms of bipolar disorder type II, hypomanic phase with irritability. He wasn't willing to commit himself quite yet, but after my second visit three days later, he recommended treatment with the mood stabilizers valproate and citalopram.

My third-year medical school wish to be a little hypomanic had been granted at last.

☞

"What did the doctor say?" Jimm wanted to know that evening.

"I don't want to talk about it," I said.

The diagnosis appealed to me. So many amazing people had bipolar disorder – Hemingway, Schumann; various writers, composers, painters. Awesome. The implications – death by suicide (Hemingway, Woolf) or from exhaustion (Schumann) – did not bother me. It was all so glamorous and romantic. In the company of geniuses, I did not care that they had ruined their lives and the lives of those around them.

"You've got a child. You need to look after yourself. You can't be staying up all night, and fighting with me, and writing articles all at the same time," Jimm badgered. "I've been taking care of Jack for weeks now. He's three years old and still not toilet-trained. I need to work. I've got deadlines and grants and patients, too. What did he say?"

"Nothing," I answered. I wasn't going to tell him that Dr. Martin thought I needed drugs even though I had already filled out the prescription.

"There's clearly something wrong with you and he said nothing?" Jimm asked. "Then you need to see somebody else!"

"One week before Christmas?!" I went into the dining room. Yanked the medicine bottles out of my purse and rattled them in his face.

"Valproate," I shouted. "Treatment for bipolar disorder type II. But guess what? I don't want to take it! I like the way I am. I can accomplish so much when I'm like this. I'm writing a grant that's going to prove how important SLOS is! A career-maker! I don't want some meds dulling me and slowing me down."

I threw the bottles across the living room – they banged on the window and clattered behind the sofa. Head tucked into his shoulders, Jimm followed their trajectory then turned back to me.

"I need to go," he said quietly. "I've put Jack to sleep. This," he gestured in the direction of the sofa, "is your decision. Yours alone." He picked up his cello case and walked out the front door – his string quartet was playing at the departmental Christmas party.

For the next two hours, I stared into the flames of our living room fireplace, the pill bottles standing sentinel behind me on the coffee table. I was interesting and interested, brilliant and productive, happy and sexy – never in my life had I felt that way. People liked me! I felt desirable, intelligent, accomplished. I was going to be a great researcher and a world-respected clinical geneticist. For the first time in my life, I loved being me, being Margaret. Jimm and Jack barred my way. Who needed them?

And yet, something inside me gave in. I swallowed the large, peach-coloured pill and the small, white oval one. I cursed, choking down the horse pill of the valproate, but I had enough sanity, enough reason left in me to realize that even though my new life was so enticing, so attractive, so glamorous, I could not sustain it.

I continued to write research papers and textbook chapters, and to knit scarves by the yard. I bought several books on bipolar disorder. I was going to become an expert on my illness by reading the entire 938-page *Manic-Depressive Illness* by Goodwin and Jamison, the ultimate authorities on the subject. Kay Jamison herself had been diagnosed with bipolar disorder type I. After about three weeks, I noticed that I had stopped ruminating on the minutiae of life. Unpleasant thoughts no longer popped into my head at all hours. The hamster wheels in my brain did not keep me awake at night. Another month passed before I stopped fighting with Jimm and shouting at Jack.

Then one day, as I walked to work on a glorious frosty February morning, I realized that I had never felt so good in my life. For as long as I could remember, something had always lurked deep within me. This dark, greedy, subconscious creature had sucked colour and flavour out of my life, rendered accomplishment and joy fake and undeserved. That wondrous and wonderful day, I noticed that the heavy feeling that had been my companion all my life was gone.

This was what normal felt like. At least for me.

I was never going to stop taking my meds.

I think of bipolar disorder type II as the poor cousin of the real McCoy: the manic-depressive illness, bipolar disorder type I. Labelled cyclothymia in the past, type II bipolar disorder delivers the same depths of depression as type I, but it never rises as high as psychotic mania. If a patient has even one episode of mania, the diagnosis automatically becomes type I bipolar disorder. As a clinical clerk at Toronto's St. Michael's Hospital, I had watched as a twenty-eight-year-old man, a scion of a prominent Toronto family, was admitted in florid mania. Thrashing against four-point leather restraints, he talked non-stop, rhyming nonsensically, swearing at everybody in the room. He had left the city four weeks earlier to begin his studies at the famed New York Film Academy and then disappeared until he was picked up by the New York police while wandering the streets of Harlem one hot and humid August night, muttering to himself. He was dishevelled and dehydrated. His family arranged for him be medevaced home. That's the typical story of mania: dancing naked on street corners, investing non-existent millions of dollars in new condominium developments, purchasing an entire drugstore's supply of rattlesnake antivenin to protect a neighbourhood from a reptile infestation only the patient is aware of. Hypomania pales in comparison – not only in the severity of symptoms but also in the damage caused to self and loved ones – and I am profoundly thankful for that. I can only imagine how I could have messed up my life had I been truly manic.

But mania is also unmistakable and easily diagnosed, and treatment can be started much earlier. Because the mood cycles in bipolar disorder type II are much milder, its diagnosis may be missed for years and may only be recognized as the severity and frequency of hypomanic episodes increases with age. Of all the upheavals and damage that bipolar disorder type II causes, the unpredictability of moods is the most difficult to bear. Along with the horrid irritability, it is the least attractive aspect of bipolar disorder type II and, together, they alienate even the most dedicated friends and the most loving relatives.

In terms of diagnosis, other disorders – much more destructive and much less treatable – are considered first, such as borderline or antisocial personality disorders, as was done in my initial hunt for treatment, when I was referred to the personality disorder specialist. And since many patients with bipolar disorder self-medicate with drugs and alcohol, their diagnosis may lay hidden under a blanket of alcoholism or drug addiction. Mercifully, I had been spared from both.

Medical treatment of bipolar disorder is one of the great success stories of twentieth-century psychiatry. When the mood stabilizing properties of lithium were discovered, US Poet Laureate Robert Lowell – also a sufferer – famously quipped, "It's terrible [...] to think that all I've suffered, and the suffering I've caused, might have arisen from the lack of a little salt in my brain."[3] Lithium allows sufferers to lead normal lives. And while many voices decry lithium as a personality killer, a stifler of creativity and genius and artistic imagination, many sufferers are profoundly relieved to be rid of the reality of the never-ending mood cycles. No genius has written anything of value during the throes of mania. And one cannot be creative when one is dead. In an outcome that is counterintuitive to all but the sufferers, suicides in bipolar disorder correspond with the upswing of

---

3   Kay Redfield Jamison, *Setting the River on Fire: A Study of Genius, Mania, and Character* (New York: Alfred A. Knopf, 2017), 184.

mood – not with depression – as patients find they simply cannot bear yet another upheaval in their life. When Virginia Woolf realized that another episode of mania was approaching, she wrote a note to her husband, loaded her coat pockets with stones and walked into the River Ouse. I thank all the gods, pagan and otherwise, that I have never been suicidal. During the depression episode in my internship, I might have thought that death might deliver me from suffering, but I had never made any plans or even talked about it.

For me, it wasn't the periods of depression that distressed me the most; it was my irritability and my unpleasantness. Lacking insight, throughout my life I had always thought that I deserved the low moods for one reason or another. I thought that they were caused by my behaviour and poor choices: I was despicable, insufferable. I pissed off classmates and teachers, psychiatrists and supervisors. First George, then Jimm and Nicolette, a dear and devoted friend, supported me through those years in spite of my mood swings and unpredictability. That they stood by me in spite of my sucking them dry like a famished vampire is testament to their patience and love and humanity and kindness – and confirmation of my enormous luck at having them in my life. They, too, suffered from my disorder.

I cherish my creativity and exuberance, but I know that they are not simply caused by the hypomania of my bipolar disorder. They are a part of me, cut from the same swatch of psychological fabric as my illness. I am creative and sensitive and bipolar, and treating my mood swings does not obliterate my creativity. At least, the medications that I take do not. I might be less likely to burst into tears in a movie theatre, but reading a beautiful story will still have me sobbing like a baby. I still laugh at a good joke and groan at bad ones. I am still the proud owner of an overactive imagination and my personality continues to fill any room I enter. I remain colourful, sometimes too colourful for my own good. The medications have not altered any of this; in fact, they have allowed me to drink it all in, to feel free to be me, to use all my talents without obsessing and worrying and pissing people off. I am much less competitive, much less bitter and a lot more easygoing than I was before being treated. I am happier.

Now that I finally knew what had been wrong with me all those years, now that I had a correct diagnosis which was eminently treatable, I just knew that this was going to be the last time that I messed up. No more pissing people off, no more anxiety and obsessing. No more depression. A normal life.

☞

One evening in early December 1999, before I started my meds, I drove to the Sydenham Lookout in Dundas. I had been driving a lot that winter, fast and without purpose, just to feel the engine roar under my foot, to see the landscape blur on either side of the road. At the lookout, I pulled into the parking and turned off the ignition. The sun had set behind my back and the black silhouettes of steel mills and chimneys laced the southern horizon, across the Burlington Basin. Lights blinked and flashed along the towers and smokestacks, along rooftops and chutes. They twinkled against the cobalt-blue sky behind them, and sparkled on the mauve and purple streaks above. Steam billowed from smokestacks as if sped onward by time-lapse photography; it fluffed, expanded, moved on. The harbour glimmered at the foot of the scene, reflecting the beauty of this spectacle of shimmering factories.

I had never realized how startlingly beautiful the Hamilton industrial skyline was; how magical, how fabulous. I stared at it until darkness fell and the panorama ahead turned into a toss of glittering diamonds across the skyline, indistinguishable from the real stars in the firmament and their reflections over the water. At that moment, the hypomanic lens rendered even the dingy, dirty industrial Hamilton harbour beautiful and important.

☞

My second research project aimed to discover how the faces of patients with Smith-Lemli-Opitz syndrome differed from the facial appearance of people without genetic conditions, the so-called "normal" people. Just as individuals with Down syndrome differ in their overall appearance, many other syndromes have a recognizable look. The medical term is "dysmorphic." Sometimes, a physician picks it up instantaneously – the same way we recognize Down syndrome, a skilled geneticist can recognize dozens of others. Sometimes, a more detailed assessment follows that instant recognition, and that's when geneticists pull out their tape measures or rulers or medical callipers and begin to measure – in fractions of millimetres – the distance between the inner corners of eyes or between pupils. They check the lengths of eye openings, the lengths and widths of ears, the height of the chin, the length of the nose. To be meaningful, those measurements are compared to the norms published in *The Handbook of Physical Measurements*, a compendium of graphs and tables of everything that can be measured on the human body, plotted against the sex and age of the patient. Even the distance between the nipples and the length of the great toe has been measured and plotted to establish such norms. The book itself is not as large as one might assume; it is a small paperback that could fit easily into the pocket of a white doctor's coat were I to wear one.

A much larger hardcover compilation, Leslie Farkas's life work, *Anthropometry of the Head and Face*, lists the norms of 132 measurements of the head and face alone, and is used by plastic surgeons to ensure that the final results of their interventions fit acceptable, eye-pleasing human norms. When I met him in 1987, Professor Farkas told me that, on the face, a fraction of a millimetre resulted in a perceptible difference in form and could make an entire face appear unbalanced. I used his book as a guide for my study, and from his long list, I chose fifteen distinct measurements to determine which, if any, gave rise to the distinct facial appearance of patients with Smith-Lemli-Opitz syndrome.

I have spent the majority of my professional life assessing human faces – fetuses, newborns, children, adults. I have seen the whole spectrum – from grotesque malformations almost unrecognizable as human to undisputed classical symmetry and beauty.

"When does a malformed fetus cease being human?" was a question posed to a genetics colleague during his interview for a genetics fellowship.

There is only one answer: "Never."

What makes a face a face? A nose, two eyes and a mouth? Children with genetic syndromes have all these requisite features, yet we recognize them as different. Sometimes it is just a matter of a minuscule difference in the spacing of their eyes, or perhaps a chin that is too far back or a tiny pit in the lower lip, but more often than not it is their overall appearance, the gestalt of their presence, that we instantly recognize as different. The human face is so much more than the sum of its parts, and a geneticist must determine if what she sees is simply a variant of normal, in keeping with the child's family resemblances or with her ethnic origin, or if it is truly outside of the norms. A face with a syndrome presents as "off" – even those without medical training can realize that the features do not add up to the expected whole. We are all able to spot somebody who is more than just unhandsome, more than simply aged or scarred. An innate part of our brain has been honed over millennia of recognizing the self of the species.

The face is a complex system. The basic structures of the facial skeleton form during the embryonic period – the first ten weeks of pregnancy – in a clockwork of countless interconnected and precisely timed steps. If the tiniest one of them goes awry, a cascade of abnormalities follows. The muscles of facial expression, buried in the subcutaneous tissues, connect the skin of the face to the bones of the facial skeleton. The muscles of the face intermingle and fuse with each other, and with the sheet of muscle at the front of the neck called the platysma. The paired facial nerves mobilize the muscles of human expression, including the muscles that circle the facial openings – the mouth and the eyes – and pucker the lips and blink the eyelids. And all of those inter-related structures need to form and grow and develop in a specific sequence to produce a face that appears normal in all of its emotional range, at rest and when smiling, crying or scowling. The smallest deviation in timing or position during the intrauterine choreography of facial development can result in a significant asymmetry or unusual expression.

"I have a staring problem," I said. The little girl giggled. Her speech development lagged and her pediatrician had referred her to me because he thought she had dysmorphic features. She sat in her mother's lap. I had been contemplating her face intently for almost half a minute before I said, "I'm not just sitting here, I'm examining her," in answer to her mother's unspoken question.

I pushed a strand of silky hair off the girl's forehead. "Let me see your pretty face." A fold of skin partly covered the inner corner of her eye and extended upward onto the root of her nose. "She has epicanthal folds bilaterally," I said.

The resident standing behind me jotted it down.

"Her forehead is tall and her eyes are normally placed. There may be a bit of hypertelorism, but it's probably within normal limits because the mother's eyes are also widely spaced. The ears," I tucked the strands of blonde hair behind the tops of the girl's pink earlobes, "are normally set and rotated and non-dysplastic. And she has a cowlick – see the hair whorl at the top of her forehead?"

The mother smiled. "Can't ever comb it flat," she said.

In spite of all the medical gibberish I had just uttered, this girl's little face did not deviate from normal and I told the mother that. Even the epicanthal folds, pleats of skin covering the inner corners of the eyes – a sign usually associated with Down syndrome – can be found in the general population. Her mother had them, too.

Because as I look at the child's features, I also examine the parents'. I can see that the shape of the nose belongs to the mother while the widely spaced eyes and long eye openings come from the dad. With cumulative features like that, sometimes a child might look dysmorphic, but in such a case it is just a confluence of familial patterns and not a genetic syndrome.

So, I stare at babies and children, and I stare at their parents. I watch the children's faces as they cry and smile, as they babble and grimace. I examine the way their hair is distributed on their skull – is the hairline too low or too high? Does it encroach onto the temples – a suggestion that the orbits may be underdeveloped? Is the hair whorl on the vertex (the exact top of the skull) or is it offset? Is it doubled? Is there one on the hairline above the forehead? I assess the shape of the ears and their position on the sides of the skull. I determine their rotation from the vertical. I examine the palate – is it roundly arched or does it resemble the ceiling of a Gothic cathedral? I shine a light into the throat to determine whether the uvula – that fleshy bit that hangs down at the back of the throat – is split or not, because a split often signifies the mildest form of cleft palate. I check the lips, nose, chin. Sometimes I measure certain distances, but more often I rely on my internal recognition of facial symmetry and arrangement. Only if in doubt do I measure and plot the result against published norms. I used to measure every feature of every patient, but with time I realized I have developed a sixth sense about it and no longer needed my measuring tape.

Sometimes, even if the child is clearly abnormal, in denial parents will insist on familial resemblance, trying to convince themselves that there is nothing wrong.

"My uncle had a tongue like that." This from a mother of a newborn with Beckwith-Wiedemann syndrome, a baby boy with a huge tongue that hung three-quarters out of his mouth. I did not contradict her; I never argue with parents about the appearance of their children. Instead, I discuss ordering the appropriate diagnostic tests. In less-obvious cases, I suggest a follow-up in a few months to see how the child "grows into her face." And many a time it happened that a child who seemed dysmorphic in the first days of life no longer appeared that way at the age of six or twelve months – and I was able to reassure the parents.

☞

Back in 2000, for the study of the facial appearance of patients with Smith-Lemli-Opitz syndrome, the measurements of the facial features had to be performed to within a fraction of a millimetre and required training. On a frosty February morning, I flew to Ottawa to train with Dr. Judith Allanson, a specialist who had previously used this methodology with several other syndromes. Judith taught me how to obtain the measurements with anthropometric instruments – spreading and sliding callipers. The ones she recommended were made in Switzerland and, like anything Swiss-made, were incredibly expensive; I had to apply for a grant from the

Hamilton Health Sciences Foundation to buy them. She also explained to me how to shoot photographs – front and profile views of the face in the Frankfort horizontal (a plane used in the measurements of the skull determined by discreet landmarks on the ear canal and the orbit). For my study, I also took photographs of the patient's whole body and close-ups of any interesting findings – ambiguous genitalia, webbed toes, cleft palates. To get better at the measurements, I practised on Jimm and Jack and whoever was willing at work – secretaries, genetic counsellors, residents. They all thought it was a hoot to have their heads and faces measured to a fraction of a millimetre.

Once I felt confident, Aleesha, Mitchell and Daniel became my first subjects. Because we knew that Aleesha would fight and struggle no matter how gentle I was, Lore agreed that I could get the measurements when Aleesha was sedated for a scheduled surgery. When my surgical colleague agreed, I marched into the operating room with my callipers. It was the fastest measurement session in the study because I didn't have to struggle with the iron will of an uncooperative toddler. In my office, Mitchell and Daniel's mom shot a series of photographs of me as I measured Mitchell's face and head so that other parents would know what the study entailed. The last image in the series – Mitchell, pouty, head slumped onto the back of an armchair, radiating joyful relief that the whole hullabaloo was over – always got a laugh. With Mitchell's photogenic if slightly unenthusiastic help, I approached patients at the next Smith-Lemli-Opitz Syndrome family conference in Detroit. The parents were happy to participate and I enrolled twenty-one patients during that June weekend.

But before that happened, I went back to Poland for the first time in twenty-one years.

9

When we left Poland at the end of August 1980, my childish plan was to return as soon as I became a Canadian citizen. Even before we left, I was counting the years 'til my return. We knew that it took three years of living in Canada to be eligible for Canadian citizenship, so I calculated I would be back in the summer of 1983. I didn't correct my calculations for the time we had to spend in Austria; in fact, while we languished there, a rumour circulated that this waiting would count toward our residency in Canada. It didn't. I had no idea about the glacial slowness of Canadian immigration bureaucracy.

We were finally granted our citizenship in July 1984, the month I received a rejection letter from every medical school I had applied to. Of course, I didn't go back to Poland then – who would? I was buried in defeat. The reality of our life in Canada was so different from the dreams we'd had in the heady days of packing, deciding what to keep and what to jettison, loading up our camper van. As we said our goodbyes to the few people who knew we were leaving and were thus burdened with keeping the secret from everybody else, we were convinced we would be victorious and accomplished. I would be a winner of scholarships and academic prizes, and my father would be a respected professional engineer with a brilliant career that people in Poland could only dream of.

☞

In the early years, with my father's unemployment, I told myself that my parents couldn't afford to send me back to Poland for a holiday, but the truth was I simply didn't want to be laughed at. Back in the '80s, what little money that we did have would still have gone a long way in Poland, but I wanted to hold my head high, proud of my accomplishments. I knew I wouldn't be able to lie; I've never been good at stretching the truth. Monika, a tween by then, did go, however. She spent two summers in

Poland, the first at a sailing camp where there were two sailboats for fifty teenagers, and the second she travelled with a Polish-Canadian scout troop and stayed with our family.

I was never embarrassed by my father's failure to get a job as a professional engineer in Canada. After he was let go from that "amazing job he got walking in from the street," and after several months of unemployment and fruitless job searches during which he felt patronized and humiliated by men younger and stupider than he, he decided to stop begging, as he put it, and took up driving an orange-and-teal Beck Taxi in the east end of Toronto. My mother, however, was mortified – an engineer with a master's degree driving a cab! My father insisted that it was only temporary. He dug in his heels and never looked back. At one point, he even managed to scrounge up enough money to buy his own cab with another driver, but that didn't last – he couldn't earn enough money both to support us and to make the loan payments. Seven months later, the partnership dissolved and the cab was sold.

In the summer of 1983, a man my father knew only slightly from work back in Poland was travelling through Canada and asked if he could stay at our place for a couple of nights. My father happily welcomed everybody into our apartment – in addition to this almost-stranger, two of his university friends, now both professors in Poland, slept in my sister's room at various times. In thanks for our hospitality, when the man returned to our hometown, he informed everybody at my father's former job where he had been such a star that Józef Nowaczyk was now driving a cab in Toronto and that my mother had to work in a toy factory to make ends meet. My mother had circulated through several small businesses where she, in order, packaged Polo perfumes and colognes, engraved brass Christmas ornaments and operated machines that knit high-end woollen ski toques. My rejections from all the medical schools only completed the dramatic picture: an utter fall from grace. I could just imagine the smirks of satisfaction at our miserable fate – schadenfreude is Poland's national pastime.

I never gave the visitor any thought, so immersed was I in my studying and my failures. But when my mother exploded, "We welcomed this viper into our house!" I had to agree with her. Then I shrugged and went back to studying. But the incident left a stain: I would not go back to Poland until I could show them all up.

When – finally – I was accepted into medical school, my first disastrous year there derailed any plans of visiting Poland. Whenever I felt better, I concentrated on building a new life in Canada, and when I wasn't doing well, I believed that I didn't deserve to go back. When I was in second-year medical school, my father was offered a job at McDonnell Douglas in Mississauga where he riveted wings on the assembly line of MD and, later, Boeing aircraft. My mother remained mortified. Two years later, he was promoted to the Boeing wing design unit and – finally – worked as a professional engineer again.

At the beginning of my third year of medical school, when I was flying high and so successful, I considered renouncing my Polish citizenship, purely for the ease and safety of travelling back to Poland. I even requested the necessary forms from the Polish Consulate in Toronto. I really wanted to go back, but I didn't feel safe, even as a dual citizen, because we had left Poland illegally and, under Communist rule, I was old enough to suffer the consequences of my parents' actions. The Canadian passport, of which I was a proud owner by then, warns dual citizenship holders that "your Canadian citizenship may not be recognized by the country of your other nationality, which may limit the ability of the Government of Canada to provide you with consular assistance." Most Canada-born individuals probably never even notice this disclaimer. Also, the Polish government demanded a reimbursement for the costs of my education to the tune of two and a half thousand American dollars. So again, I didn't go back to Poland, even though at the time I was feeling pretty great about myself.

And then, in 1989, the Berlin Wall fell. Stunned, I watched as the world I knew crumbled to pieces. Literally. No more Soviet Union? No more "bad" Germans and "good" Germans? No more "the West"? The world I grew up in was disappearing in front of my eyes, and with it, my compass. I was convinced that the changes wouldn't last, that Communism – that impenetrable, inviolate colossus – could not simply disappear but would arise again from the rubble. A year and a half later, I greeted the 1991

Moscow coup attempt with "I knew the Communists would be back." There was no way I would go to Poland during its throes of rebirth, its monetary uncertainty, its dismantling of Communism. The place was now unsafe, uncertain. Besides, I liked my new married life, my job, my financial security and my personal safety. Instead, I flew to New York City for the first time.

The summer of 1991, I saw NYC through the eyes of a child raised in Communist Poland. For many people in the Eastern Bloc, New York City was the beacon of Western civilization and culture, or – if you listened to the official propaganda – debauchery and decadence and all things wrong with the capitalist West. I never believed any of that. As I rode the Greyhound bus along the Jersey Shore, I marvelled at the perfectly straight streets crossing the island, their vistas opening onto the East River, the brilliant June sky blazing between the skyscrapers. I rode the elevator to the World Trade Center's observation deck in the South Tower and feasted my eyes on the city's expanse. I heard Ella Fitzgerald sing at Carnegie Hall in what turned out to be her last concert. I got rush seats and ended up in the last row in the highest balcony, but I didn't care – I heard Ella Fitzgerald! Live! I sauntered through the galleries at the MoMA and the Metropolitan Museum of Art, and on a blissfully quiet afternoon at the Frick Collection, I drank in Vermeer's *Mistress and Maid*. I strolled across Central Park toward the Strawberry Fields memorial and, from the pavement, looked up at the monolith of the Dakota, imagining the night John Lennon was shot there. One afternoon, as sun poured across Seventh Avenue, I lingered in a café and, imagining myself a writer in *the* cosmopolitan city, wrote what might have been a poem.

This was the place I yearned to belong to, not Poland.

☞

Two years later, in Paris for an elective rotation in metabolic diseases at Hôpital Necker-Enfants Malades, I looked up the address for the Polish Embassy in the Parisian phone book. It nestled on Rue de Talleyrand, a narrow side street of Esplanade des Invalides in the 7th arrondissement, quite the impressive address. During one of my Saturday afternoon walks,

I stared through the thick, black iron of the locked gate and, as I took in the elegant symmetry of the neoclassical structure, wondered what my life would have been like had I stayed in Poland. Deep down I knew the answer: because of my "funny spell," I would have flunked my baccalaureate and been disallowed from sitting the university entrance exams that year. Non-existent psychiatric care in Poland would have resulted in me being labelled lazy and immoral – exactly how I referred to myself at that time. I would never have been accepted into medical school, never become a pediatrician, never met Jimm. I would have lived with my mother's bitterness and nagging, with my father's disappointment at not following his dreams of a better life in Canada.

Such questions and hypothetical alternate realities dog every immigrant. Our having left Poland illegally had strengthened my commitment to making a life in Canada. After we left, there was no way back. I hadn't chosen this life for myself, but once I was here, I sure as hell was not going to compromise my dreams and plans and aspirations by meandering through a la-la land of remorse and what-could-have-been. I would have no doubts; there would be no wallowing in the past.

I shook myself and headed toward the Seine to explore the gardens of the Musée Rodin a few blocks away, my return to Poland postponed yet again.

I wanted to go back to Poland with my shield held high, not be carried on it as the Polish (borrowed from the ancient Greek) proverb says. I wanted to be a victor in the battle for a better life. Only with a great job, a university appointment, a loving husband, a beautiful son and a second baby on the way did I finally think that I had enough to show for having left. I didn't want to be pitied. I needed – wanted – accolades, recognition; to shore myself up to face what I saw as my repeated failures.

Twenty-one years after leaving, I was going back to Poland at the invitation of Professor Krajewska-Walasek, to visit the Children's Health Institute on the outskirts of Warsaw. I was going to give a lecture there and enrol Polish patients with Smith-Lemli-Opitz syndrome in my anthropometry study.

☞

At about the same time, I had reached another important milestone in my life. One day that spring, I was speaking on the phone with John Opitz, who had by that time become a friend. I was discussing a young man whom I had diagnosed with FG syndrome (yes, again). We were winding down after discussing the patient's management, and John asked in his gravelly voice, heavy and Germanic, "Do you still speak Polish?"

A beat of hesitation, followed by a flash of insight and pride. And I heard myself say, "I'm bilingual." The aptness of the word stunned me – after so many years of being ashamed and embarrassed by my accent and my linguistic deficiencies, I finally found the right word to describe myself. For the first time in my life, I owned it.

Now I was good enough to go back to Poland.

☞

For my trip to Warsaw, I chose not to fly with LOT, the Polish airlines. Partly because my father had always questioned their safety record – he used to call the Polish aircraft "flying coffins" after two of the Soviet-built aircrafts crashed in the 1980s – but mainly because I did not want to travel with a whole planeload of homeward-bound Poles. Since arriving in Canada, I had avoided my compatriots, both because I didn't want to take away from the allegiance I had made to my new country and because I didn't feel I belonged with them – some of them viewed Canada only as a temporary measure. Instead, my travel agent booked me on a flight through Paris – the cheapest business class fare she could find. I splurged on it for the first time in my life because I was twenty weeks pregnant.

From the porthole of the Air France jet, the red-tiled roofs of Polish villages and the deep emerald green of the pine forests were as familiar to me as the back of my hand. Irreplaceable and never seen anywhere else were the colours and vistas of my childhood. The spires of the small village churches piercing the skies; the bright green of the just-sprouted wheat fields; the sun-yellow of blooming rape plant; the deep, rich brown of freshly ploughed fields. The contours of farms and meadows were organic with the land – lines of roads hugged hillocks and dips in the landscape, not carved at straight angles according to a land surveyor's set square. From the sky, I followed the sinuous lines of streams, the broad shimmering ribbon of the Vistula River – that flowing silver spine of the country I had memorized poems about as a child. And as the plane banked on approach to Okęcie Airport in Warsaw and I saw the horizon of the Mazovian Plain rise to meet me, my heart skipped a beat: I was back.

Eleven years of market economy since the fall of Communism had painted the dingy grey streets that I remembered elegant pale pastels; had blanketed the previously bare city squares with restaurant patios and garden umbrellas; and had primped the clothes people wore on the streets. German- and English-made cars lined up at the lights at every corner and filled parking lots. On the hotel TV, I switched between six Polish channels – not the one and a half (one channel had broadcast only in the evenings) I had watched as a child. I saw Western European programs previously banned and the radio blared the Western stations that used to be jammed by Communist radio interference. The stores, I was soon to discover, offered foods I had never seen or tasted in Poland, and cosmetics brands I hadn't even seen in Canada. Brilliantly coloured, storeys-tall fabric billboards flapped against the facades of the few nineteenth-century Warsaw buildings that had survived the Second World War. Where in my childhood the streets were so quiet that the cawing of magpies was the loudest noise, now a cacophony assaulted my senses: street vendors hawking their wares, multi-toned car horns, sports car engines revving up at stop signs. The Poland I had left no longer existed. I wasn't back at all.

An irrational fear kept me away from Gliwice, my hometown – our old neighbours' betrayal in dispossessing us from our apartment after we had left, our furniture and books still inside, continued to sting all these years later. I had convinced myself that I would run into them were I to visit the city. And, apart from Asia, I had no friends there. And Asia was driving to Warsaw from Gliwice to meet me. She was the only person in Poland to whom I had written regular letters since leaving. From the day I met her in

1978, during the first week of high school, she had wanted to be a dentist; now, twenty years later, she had a successful practice in our hometown. She'd never married and had no children.

Asia was my first real friend. She is almost two years older than I am; she was born in April, and by the time I left Poland she had already turned sixteen and gotten her driver's licence. She was very serious and hard-working, with a mordant sense of humour; she could be a bit standoffish, a bit of a snob. I don't know how she had tolerated my impulsivity and immaturity. Because the entrance exams into dentistry were as hard as those for medical school, she had signed up for additional after-hours classes in biology and chemistry as early as grade ten. At the time, I still wanted to be an English professor. We were lucky that our parents had telephones as we talked for hours in the evenings as if we had not already covered all the news and gossip during the day. She was an only child, coddled by her parents and grandmother; I complained about my baby sister. She had lent me *The Godfather* and books of poetry by Pawlikowska-Jasnorzewska, the lyrical twentieth-century woman poet beloved by all teenage Polish girls, and I shared whatever I could from our library. She was always impeccably dressed, yet we never talked about clothes – she was above such trivial things.

Except for her hair – dyed blonde a year or two after I had left – Asia hadn't changed. She was still queenly, still elegant. I ran down the hall from my room and hugged her as she emerged from the elevator. I pulled her into my room.

"Kinda burrowish, isn't it?" she said, upper lip curling at the windows overlooking the well of a narrow five-storey courtyard. Same old Asia. She was right, of course: hardly any light reached my windows on the second floor. I elbowed her in the side.

"Next week I'm moving to the Institute's hotel," I said. "So there!"

We had brunch at Blikle's, a Warsaw landmark on Nowy Świat Street, a café I wouldn't have been able to afford when I lived in Poland: at the time it had catered to Western tourists and the prices were appropriately inflated. Afterward, we sauntered down streets lined with luxury boutiques and cafés that rivalled Toronto's Bloor Street; we loitered at art galleries and bookstores, Asia again instructing me on new books I should read. At a funky jewellery store, she approved of a thick silver choker I wanted to buy. We talked and chatted and gossiped as if I had just left Poland the day before.

But over Blikle's "American Breakfast," with orange-coloured yolks in my sunny side up eggs, I realized with sadness that Asia and I now had very little in common. We had not shared the highs and lows of the baccalaureate and university entrance exams, becoming adults, becoming doctors. She had new friends, new experiences and knowledge of which I had no part. As a wife and mother of soon to be two sons, I could not relate to her single lifestyle. Our lives had diverged on that blazing August afternoon in 1980 when my family's Fiat sedan had pulled away from the crumbling curb in front of our grey concrete apartment building. The letters we wrote informed each other of major life changes, but our camaraderie, our kinship in sharing everyday life was gone. And not having lived through martial law in Poland, "the war" as Poles referred to it, marked me as a permanent outsider to those who had suffered through it. I had missed out on the fall of Communism and the vagaries of the fledgling market economy in the 1990s – all the upheavals they had endured.

I did not belong in Poland anymore. My disorientation was dizzying.

Children's Health Institute is a tertiary pediatric hospital in a suburb of Warsaw. A referral centre for all of Poland, its construction was the brainchild of a Polish children's book author, Ewa Szelburg-Zarembina, who envisioned it as a monument to Polish children killed during the Second World War. When the Communist government approved the idea in 1968, a call went out to "all Poles, at home and abroad, and all people of good will" to participate in the building of this "significant monument" – basically a grab for immigrants' donations. In grade one, a collection can with the Centrum's logo sat on my teacher's desk. Whenever my coins clanged against its bottom, I felt a part of something special, important, something bigger than myself.

The Institute is nestled among the oaks and firs of the forests of the

Mazovian Plain; its ten-storey tower dwarfs the tallest pines. The town's name – Międzylesie, Between-Forests – reflects the Polish folk medicine belief that the microclimate of resin-scented pines and sandy soils imparts health benefits. The Institute combines state-of-the-art medical care with a sanatorium-like environment. Revolutionary for the 1970s, the Institute included a school and a hostel for parents. A physical rehabilitation wing housed gyms and a pool at a time when pools were a rare luxury in Poland. The first buildings opened their doors in May 1977. Since deciding to become a pediatrician, I'd dreamt of going there to give a talk or a lecture.

In the evenings, after I finished measuring the patients with Smith-Lemli-Opitz syndrome for my study in Professor Krajewska-Walasek's clinic, I reviewed charts, took notes and worked on papers in my room at the hostel. I took my meals in the VIP room of the cafeteria – the white china with the gold Institute logo recalling the visiting Communist dignitaries and foreign benefactors. A typical Polish dinner, a luncheon really, served at 2:00 p.m., consisted of a soup to start and a meat-and-potatoes main course, always accompanied by some sort of a pickled salad – red cabbage, shredded beets, dill pickles. For a mid-morning snack in Professor Krajewska-Walasek's office, I savoured kaiser buns with thick slabs of unsalted butter and yellow cheese washed with black currant juice. Memories carried on familiar smells and tastes flooded my consciousness.

Professor Krajewska-Walasek had been diagnosing Smith-Lemli-Opitz syndrome long before the discovery of the biochemical defect. She is an excellent diagnostician – some of the features of her patients were subtle enough to be missed. Before I arrived, she had secured institutional ethics approval for my work and had contacted her patients; six families had agreed to participate. They had travelled to Warsaw from all corners of Poland. Parents held their squirming children as I tried to measure as many features on their faces and heads as I could. They straightened dresses and shirts, and combed unruly hair for photographs. My research grant included funding for patients who had to travel to the appointment, and the parents were surprised by the one hundred and fifty złoty (equivalent of fifty Canadian dollars) I offered. Some required convincing to accept the allowance.

I savoured all of it: I loved examining the children, explaining to the parents the purpose of my study. I was learning, constantly learning, and not only genetics. My medical Polish improved with every sentence I uttered. The night before the first clinic, jet-lagged and awake until three in the morning, I had memorized as much of the Polish pediatric genetic textbook vocabulary as I could. Now, I was beginning to use it in cogent sentences.

On the first afternoon, a two-year-old boy toddled into the examining room on his gangly legs, his knees knocking together – our last patient of the day. He grinned, recognizing Professor Krajewska-Walasek, and as he did, she and I inhaled, sharply, audibly. He had a single tooth in the centre of his upper gum instead of the usual two, an unmistakable sign of holoprosencephaly, a brain malformation that had been theorized to occur in Smith-Lemli-Opitz syndrome.

Holoprosencephaly is an abnormality of the division of the brain hemispheres. When the front of the brain does not divide properly, the structures at the centre of the face also do not separate as they should. A patient may have her eyes too close together, or her nose can be very narrow (possibly only with a single nostril), or she may have a single upper central incisor. Holoprosencephaly had been theorized to occur in severely affected children with Smith-Lemli-Opitz syndrome because cholesterol is required for the activation of a developmental pathway that governs the division of the brain into its two halves. But, as with any condition, its severity extends from a lethal malformation where the brain is but a thin cyst of cortex associated with a single eye in the centre of the face and no nose to merely a single upper tooth. And here, in Professor Krajewska-Walasek's office, she and I had just diagnosed the mildest form of this anomaly in a patient with Smith-Lemli-Opitz syndrome.

I couldn't contain my enthusiasm. I asked the mother if I could photograph him, explaining much too eagerly that we had to share this finding with other doctors. Seeing the mother's dismay, Professor Krajewska-Walasek pulled me aside and told me – not unkindly – that she understood how interesting it was but that I had been overbearing. "He is her son," she said to me outside the examining room, "not a specimen." I had let my enthusiasm carry me away. She was as excited as I was – I could tell from her eyes – yet she managed to remain decorous and professional. Chastened, I stayed outside of the office as the professor spoke to the woman, probably apologizing for my behaviour. In the end, the mother signed the consent form for publication of her son's photographs.

Because many of these children had the hyperactivity typical of Smith-Lemli-Opitz syndrome, I had to find a way to examine them fast, without upsetting them or their parents. I didn't have the luxury of having them return to my office for further measurements. I didn't want to waste their time and shortchange my trip and resources, so I ended up shooting my photographs of the children's faces with a ruler held against each child's forehead, its markings and numbers clearly visible. Back in Canada, with the photos printed, I measured the facial distances on the photographs and converted them using the ruler as a scale. I also used this method for the more difficult children at the Smith-Lemli-Opitz syndrome family meeting in Detroit two months later.

There were other lessons as well. On my second day in Professor Krajewska-Walasek's clinic, I asked to examine a boy's feet and the mother began unbuttoning the fly of his corduroy pants.

"Don't worry about the pants, just take off the socks," I said.

The mother looked at me funny. "He has tights on," she said.

Tights. Of course. Suddenly my ankles and knees itched with the memory of the thick woollen tights I had always worn under my pants during sub-zero Polish winters. No snow pants or snowsuits in Poland. I had eased dozens of Canadian children out of their winter clothes in clinics and in the emergency department, and yet this difference never registered – tights and fabric pants in Poland, socks and snow pants in Canada. I explained the sartorial differences between the two countries and the mother laughed as she rolled the boy's tights down to show me her son's webbed toes.

On my last day visiting the Institute, Professor Krajewska-Walasek received a request for a consultation on a baby in the Institute's NICU – a newborn transferred from a hospital in Łódź, a city a hundred kilometres south of Warsaw. I tagged along. The NICU was no different from that at SickKids or McMaster: pinging alarms, flashing monitors, tiny bodies secured from the elements in Plexiglas aquaria, that unmistakable clean-hospital smell mixed with that of pumped breast milk and formula. The three-day-old girl we were to examine lay on a bed under bright lights and a warmer. She had six fingers on each hand and both feet ended with six toes with webbed second and third toes. We were told that behind her ribs beat a holey heart with an abnormal connection to the aorta. She had a tiny chin and a cleft palate. Not quite believing what I was seeing, I asked for an ophthalmoscope, and when I shone light into her eyes, her pupils reflected the light back whitely – she had cataracts in both. As I wheeled around to face Professor Krajewska-Walasek, we said in unison: "SLOS." What on earth were the chances that a just-born baby with Smith-Lemli-Opitz syndrome would arrive at the Institute during the four days I was visiting?

Two days later, packed in a zippy bag at the bottom of my carry-on, a tiny plastic vial with a sample of the girl's blood flew back to Hamilton with me. Within days, our molecular diagnostic laboratory found both of the mutations the girl's DNA harboured, confirmed by the Institute's molecular genetics lab. It was the first DNA diagnosis of Smith-Lemli-Opitz syndrome in Canada.

Two months after I returned from Poland, John; Lisa, a lab technician in charge of the genetic testing for Smith-Lemli-Opitz syndrome; Laura, the genetic counsellor assigned to the research study; and I attended the Smith-Lemli-Opitz syndrome family meeting in Detroit. John drove us there – I was thirty-four weeks pregnant and not allowed to fly anymore. In fact, we had a plan that if I were to go into labour during the conference, John would drive me across the Detroit River so that my baby could be born in Canada. At the conference, I gave two talks and met many parents and patients; I enrolled seventeen patients into my anthropometry study.

Although he was born ten days early, Luke did indeed wait until we'd returned to Canada. Delivered after five hours of labour and four hearty pushes, his was a completely different birth from Jack's – neither Jimm nor

I could believe how easy it was and, when it was all over, Jimm turned to me and asked, "Wanna do it again?" I replied with an emphatic "Yes!"

Luke surprised us not only with his early birth but also with a mop of almost black hair – we were expecting Jack's strawberry-blond fuzz. His cry didn't set our teeth on edge like Jack's did; it was soft and plaintive, and I immediately called him "meowy cat." The night after he was born, I sauntered into the nursery to visit him – I don't remember why he wasn't in my room – and decided to measure his head circumference. The nurses had told me he'd weighed in at 3,000 grams, which was on the 25th percentile. The paper measuring tape I stretched around his head overlapped at thirty-two centimetres and I plotted it on the newborn growth chart. It landed on the 2nd percentile. "Hmm," I thought, "his head is too small for his body." And even though "microcephalic" popped into my head, somehow the significance of that measurement did not register in my endorphin- and oxytocin-bathed brain – I was going to love him no matter what. The following morning, when I was about to start freaking out about it, our family doctor reweighed and remeasured Luke, and his head size was proportionate to his body. There was nothing wrong with him.

Over the following twenty years, I have published thirty papers on Smith-Lemli-Opitz syndrome: on its incidence in Canada and on the frequency of gene mutations in various ethnic populations around the world; on pre-natal diagnosis; and on its rare clinical features. I've consulted on patients from Vancouver to St. John's, occasionally from as far away as Hong Kong, Latvia and Cuba. With colleagues from the National Institutes of Health, we developed growth curves specific for children with Smith-Lemli-Opitz syndrome – their heights, weights and head circumferences followed distinct growth patterns, well below the norms for healthy children. Once these curves were published in a genetics journal, dieticians and nutritionists stopped berating hapless and helpless parents about their children's lagging growth, about not feeding them enough. In 2008, the Smith-Lemli-Opitz Syndrome Foundation invited me to join their scientific board. In 2012, I edited a special issue of the *American Journal of Medical Genetics* devoted to disorders of cholesterol synthesis: since the discovery of the biochemical defect in Smith-Lemli-Opitz syndrome, scientists had found other enzyme deficiencies of the pathway, and I updated the review of Smith-Lemli-Opitz syndrome in GeneReviews, the most frequently accessed online resource on genetic diseases.

I had become what I had always wanted to be: an accomplished geneticist who diagnosed and treated the rarest of diseases, an expert not only in Canada but also internationally. Yet, none of that would have happened had I not examined baby Aleesha that December afternoon in 1998 as the early winter dusk settled outside Lore's hospital room window.

☞

I don't think Lore liked me for the first several years of her daughter's life. Alecsha was in my clinic every three months; she would not gain weight and finally needed G-tube feedings: formula delivered directly to her stomach via a tube threaded through a surgical opening in her belly. Even with extra calories added to her feeds, she never reached the lowest limits for normal children – our Smith-Lemli-Opitz syndrome–specific growth curves were meant exactly for children like Aleesha. While dieticians and nutritionists insinuated that Lore didn't try hard enough, I knew the growth pattern of these children: they did not gain weight, their length lagged behind their peers, their heads stayed small. Lore spent hours every day trying to get formula into Aleesha, and Aleesha spent seconds promptly throwing it all back up. And I spent hours every month reassuring Lore that she did everything right, that as long as Aleesha continued to grow along her own growth curve – and she did – everything was fine. By the end of her first year, Aleesha's developmental delay was obvious. She did not lift her head or babble. She did not learn to walk until age five. Lore was jubilant, but I was worried – Aleesha had just become capable of getting into places where she shouldn't be, as she was without any regard for safety.

When Aleesha turned ten years old, Lore asked me whether I had known, back on that December afternoon many years earlier, that Aleesha had Smith-Lemli-Opitz syndrome even before the biochemical test had come back. I nodded.

"You're such a smarty-pants," she said. "You knew I needed those three days."

10

In the spring of 2006, in grade three, teachers at Jack's private school informed us about his worsening behaviour and learning difficulties. What we didn't know at the time, what he only told us several years later, was that he was being bullied. The teachers at the hoity-toity school didn't tell us about it, either – it was bad publicity for potential new recruits with deep pockets. As his behaviour escalated, his academic performance worsened. The principal, during a meeting that the school called, insisted on hearing tests and vision checks, as well as a battery of psychological tests and a consultation with a developmental pediatrician. It turned out that Jack had a learning disability affecting his operational short-term memory (I never figured out exactly what that meant) and scored in the "very high" IQ range, but we received few suggestions as to how to help him in school from the psychologist, teachers or principal. He was put on an individualized education plan, but the school we paid thousands of dollars for each year could not or did not want to deal with kids with difficulties. He struggled. He acted out. He did poorly academically, kids teased him and he misbehaved more. At the same time, I could see how much he wanted to belong, to have friends.

At home, he challenged everything Jimm and I said. Things got worse and worse: I screamed at him, I lost my temper; he retaliated in kind. One day, at wit's end, I slapped the side of his head, right across his right ear. The next day he complained of an earache, and when I shone a light into his ear with my otoscope, I saw a blood clot marring the pearly shine of his eardrum: the slap's pressure had broken a hair-thin blood vessel in the membrane. Guilt and shame overwhelmed me – how could I have hurt the precious little body that I had grown inside of myself with such care only a few years back? What horrible person could do such a thing?

But even that debacle didn't change my behaviour: I simply could not connect with him. I oscillated between rage at him and revulsion at myself. I apologized to him; I promised over and over again not to lose my temper only to repeat the cycle the very next day. I took my meds faithfully, I saw Dr. Martin every two weeks, I tried and tried but I could not control my anger. At school, Jack erupted when his classmates taunted him and got in trouble for his outbursts; his teachers liked him less and less.

That summer, we went to Greece for the summer holidays to visit family and to show the boys Jimm's beloved country. For weeks before flying to Athens, Jimm and I discussed how to deal with Jack and with my reactions to his temper so that we – or rather I – wouldn't blow up. In my sessions with Dr. Martin, I devised strategies. I read books on anger management. Over lunch in an Indian restaurant, Jimm wrote a list of potentially dangerous situations so that I would be able to anticipate them and talk myself down. We play-acted scenarios and situations. I can do this, I kept on telling myself, I can handle a little kid and I can handle myself. Jimm and I shook hands on it – it was our little pact. It worked for most of the trip, but one miserable afternoon had Jack and I screaming at each other on the shoulder of a dusty road near Kalamata. Jimm had pulled over in the scorching heat of the Peloponnese August, afraid to drive with a fight raging inside the car. The high afternoon sun blinded us under a pale blue sky. Luke was sobbing in the back seat – usually he would just clam up and look away when Jack and I were fighting, but this time it was too much even for our five-year-old stoic. I was holding back with all the strength I had left – I wanted to shake Jack to shut him up, to pummel him. Armed warfare raged inside of me, threatening to overwhelm me at any second. I'd had enough of his constant whining, his incessant questioning, his ongoing disobedience and his resistance to everything I said, suggested or requested. I'd had ...

"*Esy!*" The call came from a house down the road, followed by a stream of agitated Greek. A moustachioed man in a white T-shirt was shaking his fist in our direction.

Jimm began to explain in Greek and the man switched to English: "Quiet! Is quiet time. Or I call police!" He didn't care that I was about to strangle my firstborn; he was only upset that we had interrupted his siesta.

Talking rapidly in Greek, Jimm managed to mollify him. The man shrugged and clanged his gate behind him, and after a round of apologies in the car we drove onward.

☞

Back home, our tussles continued. Jack returned to private school under the jaded eyes of his teachers and I remained anxious, irritable, threatening to explode at every minute; a huge cast-iron pot, tightly lidded, with a thick liquid roiling inside and about to erupt in a plume of boiling spray. I yelled at Jack, I fought with Jimm and I wished with all my heart that somebody would call me on my actions – Jimm, Luke's nanny Jenni, even Jack's teachers. Anybody. I wanted somebody to stop me because I did not know how to stop myself. I craved accountability for what I was doing. I wasn't depressed; I was irritable and snappy and wretched. Only at work could I find some respite from the constant onslaught of Jack's moods and the demands of my home life.

I remember one Saturday afternoon rushing to drive Jack and Luke to their respective baseball practices. I sat stiffly in the driver seat, emotions swirling inside of me, threatening to drown me any moment. I clutched the steering wheel, knuckles white, and struggled to stay calm, to not give in to the tsunami coursing inside of me. I repeated to myself, "This is my life, this is my life, this is my life," over and over again. I needed to remind myself of it, needed to insist that I keep moving through it no matter what. I still choke up thinking about that day.

At the end of September, Jack saw the child psychiatrist we had been waiting to see for months. Even during that visit, Jack continued to challenge what I said until finally I snapped, "So you're saying I'm a liar?" The psychiatrist goggled at me and, at the end of the one-hour appointment, he blithely announced that Jack had oppositional defiant disorder. Until that instant, I had been living on hope – yes, hope – that Jack might have an anxiety disorder or depression because I knew that those conditions were eminently treatable with medication. But the psychiatrist – whom I remember as cold and distant, though perhaps my mood had coloured the interaction – left little room for alternatives. No, there really wasn't any treatment for it. Yes, it's quite difficult. Sorry, he couldn't help.

At home, I Googled oppositional defiant disorder: "Criminality, high rate of school drop-out, antisocial behaviour." As I kept scrolling, complications piled up. Lack of meaningful relationships. Repeated job losses. Substance abuse. Suicide. Every website – Cleveland Clinic, Mayo Clinic, American Academy of Child and Adolescent Psychiatry – said the same hopeless thing. I staggered from my computer and started to cry. I did not stop for weeks. At work, I wasted hours playing computer solitaire and *Minesweeper*. I managed to examine patients; I ordered blood tests and CT scans and brain MRIs, but I didn't check their results; I wrote chart notes, dictated letters, but those lay on my desk unedited and unsigned. No more research, no more writing articles, no more work on papers for publication.

I have no memory of how I coped at home – that time is all a grey blur of bleakness, misery and distress. Even now, trying to piece it together, I can't remember. Jimm must have taken the brunt of it, kept the peace somehow, done all the housework and child care.

When I saw Dr. Martin for my routine appointment two weeks later, he was so shocked at my appearance that he suggested hospitalization, but I convinced him that all I needed was a few days away from my family and from Jack. Before Jack's diagnosis caused the bottom to fall out of my life, I had planned to attend the American Society of Human Genetics meeting held in New Orleans that fall. It seemed the perfect break I so badly needed. With a hotel room booked, and registration and plane tickets paid for, I had nothing to lose. I would sleep and rest, lectures and scientific sessions be damned.

I never got to Louisiana. I stayed home instead. Every day, after I sent the boys to school, I lay on the living room couch and cried. I cried non-stop over my son's lost future and my own lost expectations of having a top-of-the-class, polyglot child, a Rhodes Scholar, a Harvard graduate. I cried for a son who would do all the things I had dreamed of doing myself. I cried because he was going to end up in jail or – if we were lucky – an addict living on the street. I cried so much, I sometimes wondered if I could become dehydrated from all the tears streaming down my face.

I simply could not see myself living with all my dreams trashed. I was paralyzed. I felt worthless as a mother, wretched. I was unable to do anything for my son whom I couldn't protect from his condition, from his temper, from his future. I cried day and night – not from shame or guilt but from overwhelming loss. I felt pain and sorrow and hopelessness.

After a week of this nightmare, Jimm insisted I see Dr. Martin again. This time, I sat hunched in his private office, motionless, tears streaming down my cheeks. I could not meet his eye – just a week earlier I had pulled off the scam of the century, convincing him that I only needed a short holiday while in fact I was profoundly depressed, the most depressed I had ever been. My difficulties with Jack only deepened the low mood that had been smouldering since the summer. Dr. Martin took one look at me, picked up his phone and, after a short conversation I couldn't follow, told me that there was a bed available the next day at Homewood, a psychiatric hospital and treatment facility in Guelph. It was mine if I wanted it.

I wanted it.

☞

On October 13 – a Friday, fittingly – Jimm drove me to Guelph. Jack and Luke were at school and were spared the sight of my leaving, my cheeks soaked with tears yet again. When I climbed into our navy blue Acura, I was so flummoxed Jimm had to help me with the seatbelt. I sobbed the whole way there, wiping my cheeks and the snot from my nose on the sleeve of my fleece jacket. I had no idea that Jimm was scheduled to give a keynote lecture at a national conference in Hamilton that afternoon, and even if I had known, I wouldn't, couldn't have cared. I didn't even register the speed with which he bombed north on Highway 6. The overcast sky threatened rain, but not a drop fell as we sped past the blurred red-orange foliage. In less than half an hour, he pulled up to the curb at Homewood's main entrance.

"I need to get back," he said. "Are you going to be okay?"

It didn't even occur to me that he could have stayed – I knew he had work to do, our kids to look after. I nodded. I could do this. I wanted to do this. It was my only hope.

The entrance to Homewood was in the '60s-style one-storey wing that connected to the historic structures behind it. Beyond, tall trees scratched at the sky. Five concrete steps spanned the side of the building and led up to a double door. Clusters of men and women of all ages and body types stood around puffing on cigarettes, their collars up against the cold. Apologizing yet again, Jimm peeled away from the curb. He made it back in time, he told me weeks later, but had no recollection of the drive.

I don't remember going in and finding the admissions desk, but I must have, because soon I was sitting in a tiny bare room, facing a clerk typing my information into her desktop computer. Her kind eyes watched me as I sobbed through the interview and answered in monosyllables. Only one of her questions – "Have you ever committed arson?" – shocked me enough to lift my head and make eye contact with another human for the first time in over two weeks. She shrugged.

"It's on the list," she said. "I have to ask."

Wow, said a little voice in my head. This is for real – I'm being admitted to a psychiatric ward where questions about arson are routine. The implication of criminality did not register in my addled mind at the time.

At the end, the admitting clerk asked for my credit card. The only available bed was in a single room and my insurance did not cover private accommodation. Even in my stupor, I realized how lucky I was to be able to just put down my Visa and pay for it. I briefly wondered what would have happened if I couldn't pay. Would they send me out into the cold the way I was, crying and snot-nosed?

The clerk tore a strip of paper from a computer printout and slipped it into a bright orange plastic case she clipped onto my right wrist: my name, date of birth, hospital number. After she snipped the extra plastic off with scissors, she locked them back into her drawer. I stared at the slip on my wrist and remembered the last time I had one: when I gave birth to Luke, five years earlier.

Paperwork completed, she picked up the phone and told whoever was on the other end that she was bringing me upstairs.

"No, I should," she told the person on the other end. "She's in no shape to find her way on her own."

"Thank you," I said. Or at least I hope I did; I don't really remember.

I do remember the door to the ward. "MacKenzie II" was stencilled on the chicken wire–reinforced glass panel. The clerk pushed a button next to the door. The door buzzed, and when she pulled it open, I stepped into a psychiatric ward for the first time as a patient. A brightly lit corridor stretched the length of the building and a black wall phone hung at its far end. Doors opened on either side, most of them patient rooms with two beds, but one, on my left, was crowded with three beds arranged in parallel. A woman with gorgeous red hair laid on the middle one, reading a book; a large stuffed white bunny on the bed next to her was covered with a granny square afghan. The glassed-in nurses' station, until now my domain in every hospital ward, was out of bounds. A corridor branched off to the left, ending in what looked like a lounge. Bare walls. Polished, beige linoleum reflected the fluorescent ceiling lights.

A nurse named Glen met me at the nurses' station and showed me a room as nondescript as he: a grey linoleum-lined square with a single hospital bed in the middle, a metal-legged plastic chair beside a taupe wall, a single-door closet and a small wall desk, both covered in cheap-looking plastic oak facsimile. A floor lamp listed in the corner. A window opened onto an inside corner of the yard where two wings converged; it abutted a brick wall on the left and, facing it, branches of a tall sugar maple tree hung inches from the glass pane. After I locked my bag in the closet, Glen walked me around the ward: he showed me the showers, the washroom with a tub, the toilets; the clean utility room where bedsheets, blankets and thin towels were stacked on wire shelves. These would come in handy, I realized, since I had brought nothing with me except for my wallet. The common room had a small boxy TV in the corner and institutional quilts on the wall; on one side, windows looked out over the street Jimm had just driven up, and in the other direction over the square of browned lawn I had noticed through my room's window. People curled on the sofas and in armchairs. *The Young and the Restless* flickered on the screen, adding to the air of lassitude and torpor. In the hallway, we passed a middle-aged yet completely grey-haired woman banging her walker on each side as she zigzagged from wall to wall, apparently unable to walk straight – "Fuck" erupted from her mouth every time her walker veered off course.

After Glen left me in my room, I paced the four yards of the floor beside my bed like a caged lynx, moaning, "Jack, Jack" for about an hour until Glen returned to take me to meet the attending psychiatrist. After a brief interview during which Dr. Lysak ascertained, from between my sobs, who I was and why I was there, she prescribed an urgent dose of Seroquel, a newly introduced antipsychotic tranquilizer that was also found to help with depressive episodes of bipolar disorder. Glen went to get it. Within half an hour of gulping it down, I stopped crying and decided that I could handle it here. I would stay away from Jack for a couple of weeks, get better and figure out how to deal with him. It was going to be fine. After weeks of agony and worry and crying, it was a welcome relief. Nothing to worry about! I felt light as a feather, a Seroquel-induced miracle. I did not care that the succour was pharmacological – I needed it after all those anguish-filled weeks.

I fell asleep even before lights out at 10:00 p.m. I vaguely remember a flashlight shining into my room when the nurse checked in on me, a procedure I remembered from my psychiatry rotations, but each time I rolled over and went back to a dreamless sleep.

The following morning, a Saturday, I woke up to the low murmurs of patients lined up in the corridor outside the door to my room. They were queuing for their morning meds at the dispensary window of the nurses' station directly across the hall. After I swallowed my white pills, the oval citalopram and the round Seroquel, I lay on the bed in my room, door ajar as required (ward rules), nothing to do except think of my predicament. But the Seroquel made it all acceptable, bearable. I watched the brown leaves on skeletal branches outside my window hanging on for dear life as the wind whipped them around, and I remembered a story I had read as a child: A tubercular girl on the verge of death told her mother that she would die when the last leaf fell off the vine outside their basement window. Every day when she woke, she glanced through the window, the leaves falling until only a single bright yellow leaf remained. She was ready. But that lone leaf weathered November thunderstorms and December snow-falls, holding tightly onto its stem. In the new year, when even the frosts didn't tear the leaf down, the mother realized that the girl was getting better. It wasn't until they ventured outside after the spring rains that they saw the yellow leaf had been painted onto the dirty stucco, most likely by the elderly painter who had lived in the rooms next to theirs but who had died from pneumonia during the winter.

Somewhat melodramatically, I wondered where I would be when the last leaf fell off the branch outside *my* window.

Jimm visited that afternoon. He had left the boys with our nanny and brought me a care package: flaxseed crackers and Gorgonzola, tangerines and green grapes, Lindt chocolate and three large green bottles of San Pellegrino. "This psych hospitalization wasn't so bad," flashed through my mind, even though I realized that he had gone overboard. He looked uncomfortable and kept on asking me if I was okay. He stroked my hair and told me it was going to be all right, that he was proud of me for doing this difficult thing, that the boys would be okay, that he appreciated what I was doing for all of us. He looked so worried I didn't have the heart to tell him that I was feeling better already, courtesy of my meds and being away from the children and work.

Because being in the hospital was such a relief.

I didn't care who knew of my hospitalization, my depression or my bipolar disorder. I was not mortified, I was not embarrassed, I was not humiliated. I was sick. I needed help and that was all I could think about. I hoped somebody would finally help me deal with Jack or, rather, with my feelings about Jack even though I was convinced his situation was hopeless. That was how I had interpreted the results of my web search, the DSM-IV entry, all the articles I had read. I knew there would be no cure, that oppositional defiant disorder was for life. Jack would never change and it would be entirely up to me to learn to live with his failures and temper and outbursts. I wanted to love him in spite of all this; I did love him in spite of all this – but I was destroyed by his supposed diagnosis and the future I thought it spelled out for him.

And I wanted to say to those who knew me at my worst: See, I'm not a bad person. I'm not vile, not wicked, not immoral. As long as I stayed at work and at home, I was just an awful, miserable person without a shred of patience, but my depression offered an explanation for my behaviour. I wondered, though: Was I still a terrible mother?

I hoped that I would learn to accept Jack for who he was, and learn to accept myself as his loving, flawed mother. I hoped somebody could persuade me that it was not my fault, that I didn't cause any of this to happen, that I hadn't failed as a mother because I never followed through with *1-2-3 Magic* or *The Explosive Child*, books I had read and tried to use to help him but gave up on because it was all too much and too difficult. I knew I hadn't done everything I could have done for him – I hadn't taught him how to control his anger, even though Jimm and I did enrol with him in a "Temper Tamers" program. Somehow, we just never could follow any of its recommendations consistently. I didn't teach him how to behave properly at school and at sports. I did not explain it all to Jimm so that he could follow the recommendations and directions. It was all my fault.

I saw so much of the child me in Jack. I had never been good at making or keeping friends, and I unthinkingly pissed off classmates and teachers at school almost every day. One day, I had lugged a heavy encyclopedia to school to prove to my teacher that the sun was a star and not a planet, as she had claimed in class. In the elementary school world atlas we all bought – a folio-size, soft-covered booklet of twenty-eight pages – the inside of its back cover presented a diagram entitled "The Planets of Our Solar System." This was the source of my teacher's and classmates' knowledge of the universe, and on it, the sun, drawn to scale, edged the left side. But my father's love for astronomy had rubbed off on me and I couldn't stand people being wrong. Also, I loved being right. The morning I brought the encyclopedia to school, my teacher's grimace hovered high above my head as she ordered me to take my place. From then on, she complained that I couldn't sit still, that I had no manners, that I disobeyed her orders. Almost every day brought a new warning in my communication booklet, and almost every week my mother had to report to school for "a chat" with her.

Other teachers were more sanguine about my antics, probably because of my good marks. But I remained a semi-outcast for most of my school years in Poland, a situation made worse on arrival in Canada. No wonder I didn't know how to socialize my son. And I, too, had trouble controlling my temper, even as an adult. It *was* my fault: first, in giving Jack my crummy genes; and second, in not teaching him how to overcome them. I deserved to be in Homewood. I deserved to feel wretched. I deserved the misery and shame, the stigma and the pity. I had brought it all on myself and then inflicted it on my son. In spite of my love, Jack never had a chance. And now, the time had come for the universe to pay me back.

The nurses' notes from my first two weeks post-admission read, repeatedly: "teary, flat affect, overwhelmed with thoughts about son"; "very negative, pessimistic"; "restricted affect"; "sad, occasional smile." That sounds about right. But in spite of the hopelessness and the crying, I also began to feel a glimmer of light – I was here, I was going to work the hardest I could at getting better and I would get back to normal eventually. I stupidly – yet wholly – believed that this would be the last time, that hospitalization and hard work would fix me for good, finally. I would be normal. I wanted to work so hard that I would impress the nurses and therapists, even the psychiatrist. And I wanted to prove that Dr. Martin was right in sending me here. I would not betray the trust he put in me. I was going to be the best patient they had – whatever that meant. Well, at least the one working the hardest at getting better. Just show me what to do and I would follow it to a T.

At Homewood, patients were not allowed to have laptops and cellphones. I could check my email in the library, on a desktop computer that to use, I had to sign up on a clipboard tied to it with white rope, but I received very few emails. Ron Carter, my boss at the time and a kind and caring man with a tendency for pessimistic exaggeration, had sent an email to all of my coworkers: "Margaret's family would appreciate space and consideration at this difficult time." I had never asked for it, neither had Jimm. But everybody at work took his injunction to heart and I received no emails, not even get-well wishes. But Ron did send a bouquet of flowers the size of a sheaf of wheat, and Susan and my secretary sent me an ultra-soft navy blue blanket and hot-pink fuzzy slippers. I wore the slippers with my big hooded fleece jacket every day. The jacket hung down to my thighs and had huge sleeves I could burrow into and disappear. Its combination of pinks, reds, oranges and turquoise made my eyes water if I looked at it for too long, but I pretended that it cheered me up, even though nothing did, nothing could.

When my misery began to lift with the Seroquel, all I wanted to do was work at getting better. When I received my schedule for the next two weeks, I got upset, angry almost, that I had not been signed up for art therapy. I had already heard from other patients how helpful it had been to them. I wanted the best; I wanted to get going full speed to recovery; I wanted to work, work, work, sleeves rolled up, ready to battle my demons in all ways possible. And here, a glitch in the schedule was already slowing me down. The charge nurse explained that the next sessions started in only two weeks and that I was already registered for it. I calmed down.

"And you'll be busy enough with your other sessions," she added.

My schedule did not look busy at all. Twice a week a group session on cognitive behavioural therapy, weekly horticultural therapy, pottery – or was it ceramics? We didn't throw clay; we only painted and glazed already-formed vases, plates and jugs. There was a women's group on the ward and optional 8:00 a.m. walks in the Homewood gardens with the recreational therapist. What would all these accomplish? With only one session a week with Dr. Lysak, it seemed that little was specifically tailored to me, to my needs, to my misery. With only group this and group that, how was I to get better?

Since that schedule failed to fill all of my time, I scoured the Homewood library for self-help books. One, *When Anger Hurts Your Kids*, seemed written expressly for me. I worked through all of its exercises, identifying "red-hot trigger" thoughts, their magnifiers and labelling. I worked through actual situations such as doing homework or getting Jack ready for hockey. Another book, *How to Control Your Anger before It Controls You*, suggested that I describe the anger driving the bus of my life. I wrote:

Short, beefy (...) guy with a short neck with bulging veins. Also veins on his forehead and hands tightly clenched on the steering wheel – just you wait if you think he will let anybody near it! His knuckles are white from tightening them; his hands are hairy. Has small, beady eyes, deep set and mad-looking. B/c he is so short, his feet barely touch the pedals, he has to sit at the edge of the driver's seat. Just a little bit of hair around his ears, oily and stuck to his bald skull. Being out of control of my anger life feels hopeless, sad and fearful as well as angry! I want it back!

I have no idea where he came from, this embodiment of my anger, a driver in the midst of a steroid road rage.

My graphomania resurfaced. In my poppy seed–like handwriting, I answered questions in the self-help books, hoping to write away the pain and feelings of failure. This writing also uncovered my problems with envy, self-esteem and constant comparing to others that had been there all along, but I was finally naming these beasts for what they were. Within two weeks, at the table in the Homewood library, I had covered an entire pad of white, pale blue–lined paper with a red margin on the left. I wrote a letter to Jack to apologize for what I had done and to tell him how much I loved him. I scribbled and scribbled in the hope of solving my problems. If only it were enough.

On the Tuesday morning of my third week there, I sat down for a session with Mary, the social worker assigned to my case. When she asked me whether I had ever hurt my children, I admitted that I had hit Jack that one time.

"I'll have to report it to Children's Aid," she said.

Anger, fear and shame flooded me. No! I slammed the desk with both palms. "You can't!" I shouted.

Mary jumped in her seat, eyes popping wide as she swivelled to glance at the door, probably wondering if she was safe alone in the room with me.

I was mortified. I had done it again, all my hard work down the drain. I had just proved to her that I was still unable to control my anger. What a mess. I started to cry. Back home, I *had* wanted somebody to call me on my behaviours. Now, with me at Homewood, knowing that the boys were safe, that it was not going to happen again, there was no need to call Children's Aid. Except that it just did happen again. I couldn't bear the shame of the teachers at Jack's school knowing it all – my hurting him, Children's Aid investigating – as if Jack hadn't suffered there enough already. I pleaded with Mary, knowing full well that she was legally bound to report any potential danger to my children. Alone in my room, I sobbed, curled up in bed for the rest of the morning.

Shame overwhelmed me, but after I settled down, I resigned myself to the investigation: it was the right thing to do for my sons. My shame and humiliation did not matter. In the end, the agency visited our house and interviewed Jimm, Jenni and the boys but did not contact the school – a small mercy. The Children's Aid social worker notified Homewood that she planned to visit again after I returned home, to ensure that there was no danger to my sons, and requested a report from the psychiatrists when I was discharged.

Jimm met the hospital team involved in my care during my second week there. After Dr. Lysak discussed the plan and the medication changes, and my current mental shape, Jimm thanked everybody for taking such good care of me. Then he asked how much longer I would have to stay.

"At least three more weeks," Dr Lysak answered. "That way Margaret will be able to benefit from all the programs she's attending." Jimm's body sagged like a trench coat hung from a peg in the wall. He really wasn't expecting that and neither was I. If Dr. Martin had told me that it would be five or six weeks, I would have never agreed to go to Homewood – no way could I expect Jimm to fly solo for such a long time, even with the nanny's help. But now that I was there, now that I was feeling like I was getting better, I wanted to stay. I wanted to finish the work I had started.

At Homewood, I had the luxury of time, to devote myself to getting better and to not worry about Jack, the house, work or academia. I got a full night's sleep every night, I went for a walk on the grounds three times a week with a recreational therapist and used a treadmill the other days.

I could devote time to figuring things out: my anger, my frustrations, my distorted thinking patterns, the latter aided by group sessions in cognitive behavioural therapy. I enjoyed art therapy, where I produced collages of perfect home life cut out from colour magazines; I fussed with my plant arrangements in the greenhouse. I don't know how these helped, exactly, but they balanced and calmed me, and thus allowed me to do the hard work of reshaping my thinking about Jack and my attitudes toward work. Even my home visits on the weekend, the so-called "therapeutic leaves," were an opportunity for therapeutic work. Glen debriefed me on Monday mornings.

I am ashamed to admit it, but even after the team meeting, I didn't give much thought to how Jimm was coping at home. At first, I was too stunned, too anguished, too sick to think about anything other than my own pain. I was misery incarnate, one big hunk of wretchedness and pain, my brain consumed by loss and hopelessness. I had no brain capacity left to think about anybody or anything else. And after the Seroquel started to work its magic, when the black fog began to lift, I was so relieved to be getting better that I simply relished the dark cloud lifting from my mind, my spine straightening and shoulders sliding down my back, my tears not pouring out anymore.

But while I enjoyed uninterrupted sleeps, Jimm was getting up every night to tend to Luke's cries. Before breakfast, I strolled in the Homewood gardens on the Eramosa River or walked the labyrinth as he struggled to get the kids out of bed and dressed and fed and ready for school. I sat in group therapy or taught myself meditation and relaxation while he ran from clinic to ward and back again, attending patients and struggling to write grant applications and research papers – he would never ask for a leave of absence from work for any reason. I watched TV and knitted a vest for my father in the evenings as Jimm fought with Jack over homework and calmed Luke's tantrums. I could go to bed any time I wanted while he struggled with the nighttime routines. He shopped for groceries, cooked dinners, cleaned the kitchen, spent whole weekends alone entertaining the boys. Neither my mother nor his brother or his brother's wife ever helped; my father – who would have – was travelling in Poland for eight weeks, and my sister had moved to the Far East by then. I have no idea how Jimm did it. The nanny was there in the afternoons but not available on weekends, and our wonderful cleaning lady cleaned the house spotless every Wednesday – that was all the help he had. He told me much, much later that all he remembered of that time was bone-wearying fatigue and sadness. He couldn't even play his cello – there wasn't enough left of him for that.

"One night, I sat down on the steps outside Luke's room waiting for him to fall asleep," he told me much later, "and I didn't think I would ever get up." But he did, and did it again and again for five weeks.

Because that's how long I stayed in Homewood: five weeks to the day. By the time I left, fall was long gone and I hadn't even noticed the last leaf falling off the branch outside my window.

The week before I was supposed to go home, Jimm came to Homewood for the discharge planning meeting. My whole team was there: Dr. Lysak, Glen, Mary, even the recreational therapist. Before anybody had a chance to say anything, Jimm stood up and thanked them all for the excellent care I had received. He said that he could see already how much better I was doing. And how grateful he and the boys were for all the help I had received. He never mentioned how hard it was for him.

"Will I be able to go back to work when I get back?" I asked.

"I wouldn't recommend it," Dr. Lysak said. "The holidays are coming, with all their stresses. I suggest at least three months to get used to being back home. For everybody's sake."

Four months off work. How would I explain this to Ron Carter? Our other geneticist had accepted a position in Calgary before I was hospitalized so there was no clinical geneticist at McMaster, no geneticist doing prenatal – it was all provided by obstetricians with no physician to supervise the genetic counsellors the whole time I had been at Homewood. Basically, with my hospitalization, our little department folded. I felt awful about it.

But I wasn't going to argue with my psychiatrist before my discharge.

☞

At home, I felt fragile, uncertain. I was terrified of losing my temper with Jack, of fighting with Jimm. I worried that any progress I had made would evaporate the first time Jack challenged me. Every day that I didn't blow up was a victory, a sign that things would get better. The Children's Aid worker came for a house visit and signed off on our case. On a Saturday two weeks after my coming home, Jimm drove all of us to the Birks store at Toronto Eaton Centre, and he and the boys chose a two-string pearl necklace for me. "To show you how much we appreciate all that you did for us," he said when he presented it to me. He really believed that going to Homewood was a huge sacrifice for me and not self-preservation. I had tried to explain it to him but still he insisted on my bravery and dedication, so I stopped.

Christmas came and went without any glitches. After New Year's, I began to plan my return to work. I wasn't ashamed or embarrassed about my hospitalization – on the contrary, I was proud that I had gotten better, and I looked forward to going back. I felt happy and hopeful.

This really was going to be the last time I faltered.

11.

All the writing I did at Homewood reminded me that once upon a time I had wanted to be a writer. Shortly after we were married, sixteen years earlier, I had whispered to Jimm those exact words: "I want to be a writer."

"Why are you whispering?" Jimm asked. He sounded annoyed, but I didn't dare say it out loud – it seemed too presumptuous, too daring to even wish for let alone say out loud. Writers were rarefied beings who sojourned on a different plane of existence. How dare I aspire to be one of them?

I loved seeing my name in print upon publication of my first medical article. Since then, my writing had been hijacked by academic pursuits, but my love of putting words on paper remained. I preferred writing case reports, the mainstay of clinical genetics research: single-patient stories of disease, a recounting of a life with rare or until-then-unknown conditions. So even as I pursued my medical career, I had been telling stories. Case reports are considered the lowest form of clinical research, but I churned out so many that my colleagues dubbed me "the queen of case reports."

In Homewood, a leisure therapist suggested journaling as something I might want to explore. I disliked the term immediately – I detest verbing nouns. Wasn't journaling simply keeping a diary? Writing in a journal? Except that in the context of self-help, journaling refers to the practice of writing specifically to identify bothersome thoughts and beliefs, and to alleviate stress. Is that why I had kept a diary as a girl? Why I had written all those long letters to Asia? Was there an emotional reason behind my lifelong hypergraphia?

In 1997, feeling settled in my career at McMaster, I had leafed through its Continuing Education calendar. It offered a creative writing diploma with a solid selection of courses. I decided to register for it once I'd established myself, when my academic rat race had ended. With a steady job and regular hours, I would be able to carve out time for writing, I had thought.

But the carrot of academic promotion dangled in front of my nose, and I found myself enjoying my new job so much I soon forgot about writing anything other than medical papers. Occasionally, I would think about writing fiction – I had always wanted to write short stories; novels were totally beyond my reach – once I reached the rank of associate professor. Then my research took off and Luke was born, and during that maternity leave I became obsessed with genealogy.

For two years, I learned the principles of genealogical research and proof. For hours, I stared at microfilms in the local Family History Library, tracking my peasant ancestors back in time. Locating long-dead great-great-grandparents turned out to be easier than I had initially thought. Once I identified the parish to which their hamlets belonged, it was only a matter of locating the appropriate microfilm and spending hours reading pages and pages of old parish books. I managed to track my oldest ancestor to 1688, to a tiny Silesian hamlet only thirty kilometres from Gliwice, the city where I had lived before we left Poland. I never knew that my father's grandmother had come from there and neither did he. And while my mother discouraged and actively sabotaged my interest in her progenitors, for reasons she never shared other than "Don't dwell on the past, look to the future," my father cheered for every new generation I unearthed.

I discovered a lively online community of Polish genealogical hobbyists, and after several months of answering their questions based on the knowledge I had gleaned from English-language genealogy textbooks and guides, I decided to write a how-to book on genealogy in Polish. Until then, the only genealogy publications in Polish were devoted to tracking nobility and to heraldry. My book, *Searching for Ancestors, Genealogy for Everyone,* three hundred and fifty pages hardcover, was published in 2005 by Państwowy Instytut Wydawniczy, a venerable Polish publishing house founded in 1946. It became a bestseller in Poland and made me a minor celebrity in Polish genealogical circles. But it wasn't this success that delighted me; rather, as I was writing it, I had an almost physical feeling of pleasure in using a hereto fallow part of my brain, this new pursuit was so different from my usual science- and evidence-based studies and writing. It wasn't creative writing, it wasn't literary, yet it still felt totally different than writing medical papers and articles and grants – a combination of freedom and discovery. I loved that feeling. I wasn't simply regurgitating facts and producing formulaic case reports or review articles in the well-trodden ruts of academic writing; I was creating something new.

My book was centred around cases from my own research that illustrated how to solve some of the more difficult problems I had faced, those brick walls of genealogical research – an approach that in the teaching of clinical medicine is called problem-based learning. I managed to combine my two loves: genealogy and medicine. I studied Polish history and geography, deciphered Latin and German handwriting in parish books, and learned the vocabulary of genealogical notations and ancestor numbering systems. I particularly enjoyed decoding the *morbus* – causes of death – rubric in parish records as I tried to figure out to what modern diseases those ancient descriptors referred to. I never thought of myself as a writer, simply as a teacher writing a textbook, but at the same time, I found myself imagining my ancestors: huddled in their thatched smoke-filled huts in winter, toiling over back-breaking field work in spring, harvesting wheat and loading hay onto the manor lords' horse-drawn drays in late summer.

All of my ancestors were peasants and, until the 1864 emancipation, were mostly indentured serfs treated as chattel by their landed gentry masters. They were sold when their hamlets were sold, flogged and whipped for the smallest offences. Until my father's generation, they barely had primary school education, and before the twentieth century, they were illiterate. But in the bare-bones notes about their lives – records of birth, marriage, death – I looked for personality; for their connections with me, their direct descendant. My favourite ancestor, the one who stirred my imagination the most, is Józefa Koperek, my great-great-grandmother on my father's side. Born in 1817, she was married at the age of sixteen and gave birth to five children, three of whom – along with her husband – she buried during a cholera epidemic in 1852. She married again, a man fourteen years her junior, and gave birth to my great-grandfather at the age of forty-one. She buried her second husband shortly thereafter only to marry for a third time. She outlived her third husband (!) and died at the age seventy-four. I like to think of her as a tough and wise woman who knew her worth even within the still-feudal society. I wondered what parts of her lived on in me – was I as tough as she was? I threw my knowledge of genetics into the pot and had a blast imagining the infinitesimal-yet-real threads connecting us across continents and centuries – the nanoscopic unbroken threads of DNA.

When I wrote my genealogy book, I did not consider myself a writer. I simply collected information and presented it in an approachable manner. It was teaching, it wasn't writing. My writing wasn't literary. My writing wasn't fiction.

And I wanted to be such a writer.

Unfortunately, by the time I returned from Homewood, McMaster University was phasing out its creative writing program. Only two courses remained on offer in the winter term of 2007. I enrolled in Finding Your Voice – an introduction to creative writing. From January to April, every Thursday afternoon I signed off to my genetic counsellor, and from two until four thirty, I learned how to write.

The poet Catherine Graham taught this group: several retired-women-who-wanted-to-write-memoirs, a timid twentysomething man, an eccentric ex-hippie, a grey-haired grandfather and me. Catherine was a very, very good teacher who, with quiet authority, led us through prompts and the reading of some outrageous writing – not all of it mine. I wrote about the Silesian lace that spilled from the laps of my nanny and her cronies as they crocheted tablecloths, curtains and pillowcases from blindingly white, gossamer-thin cotton thread. I wrote about the clouds abutting the hills I visited with my father around the Polish hamlet where one of my great-grandmothers was born. I wrote about the soughing of the soaring Baltic pines swaying above as I traipsed through forbidden dunes on the summer holidays of my childhood; about the starry scar of my belly button. Incredibly, I was crafting sentences in English, savouring its words, building stories in space where before there had only been blankness and vacuum, emptiness and loss. I was excavating emotions and dressing them in words and phrases, giving them form. It was such a rush – I found myself able to communicate joy and delight, pain and sorrow. And as I read out loud in class what I had written, I felt I was finally being heard.

As I completed class assignments, I revelled in putting words together to make sense of my inner workings, to understand the mess that were my feelings, jumbled and painful. I found words for the morass of emotions that either choked me or threatened to spew forth at the slightest provocation. I pored over dictionaries and a thesaurus, wrote long lists of synonyms, copied definitions. My English vocabulary expanded in a way I hadn't experienced since those first heady months of medical school when we were learning a whole new language called medical English. *The Oxford English Dictionary* contains over a million entries and, word by word, I made glacially slow progress into its riches.

Over the years, as I progressed in writing fiction, first on my own and then for my Master of Fine Arts program, which I began in 2014, certain themes held me prisoner: how a genetic mutation, a single spelling change in the DNA, altered a person's life irrevocably; how ruthless and unfeeling genes were (I anthropomorphized them, saw them as obnoxious imps dancing on DNA strands); how prenatal life-and-death decisions overburdened me and how responsible I felt. I didn't think of it as therapeutic; I simply wanted to be a writer, an artist. For a long time, I shied away from writing non-fiction because it was too raw, and bestowing my emotions upon fictional characters gave me the distance I needed to process them. But I couldn't find answers in fiction, which was why I began writing creative non-fiction: about my genealogical research and a trip I took with my sons to Horyniec, my grandmother's birthplace; about *Polynésie, la mer*, a Matisse cut-out of underwater creatures; about translating myself into English.

And I wrote about Savannah.

12

Nine years before I began that first writing class, I had been called in to see a couple in the prenatal diagnosis clinic. "Abnormal bones" was all the referral note had said. Shannon was nineteen weeks pregnant. Her fetus had a long skull with a tall, narrow forehead. The brain inside appeared normal, but the baby's arm and leg bones were bowed and three weeks behind schedule in length. By the time Shannon was twenty-four weeks pregnant, these bones lagged eight weeks behind and the ribs did not extend all the way around the chest. The heart of the baby filled the entire chest cavity and left no room for the lungs to grow. In the womb, the breathing movements of the baby draw the amniotic fluid into the lungs and the liquid stretches the developing alveoli, the tiny air sacs where oxygen is transferred into the blood. If anything interferes with this process, the overall lung area will be too small for adequate gas exchange and, when finally breathing on its own after birth, the baby will essentially suffocate. In the case of Shannon's baby, it was the smallness of the rib cage, the shortness of the ribs, that was stunting the growth of the baby's lungs. Powerless in the face of physiology, there was nothing that we could do to fix it.

The radiologist, the consulting neonatologist and I all agreed the baby's lung surface would likely be too small to sustain life. And I thought: Maybe this baby should not be born? Reluctant to deliver terrible news yet again, I dragged myself into the consultation room.

"I don't care if she's in a wheelchair," Shannon said before I even had a chance to explain anything about the baby's chest. "I don't care if she's crippled. I don't care if she's retarded. We will love her anyway." Fat tears meandered down her cheeks and dripped off her jaw, dotting the pale green T-shirt stretched taut over her pregnant belly.

"It's not so much the legs and the arms," I said. "It's the ribs and the size of her chest. If her ribs are too short, her lungs won't grow, and they won't be big enough for her to breathe."

"How do you know?" Shane, the father, asked.

"She may need a breathing tube when she's born," I said. "She may need a ventilator to breathe for her. And we don't know how long she'll need it for."

"So, there *is* something that you can do." Shannon's eyes widened.

"If we put her on a ventilator, she may need to stay on it for the rest of her life ..." I began.

"You can help her," Shannon breathed.

She missed my point entirely.

There was one last question that I had to ask. "In situations like this, some parents may want to consider ..." I said, wishing Shannon would hear what I had said and was continuing to say about the lungs, the danger of her baby's condition. I didn't even finish my question – Shannon said, "No! I'd never do anything like that."

"We'll support any decision you make," I said. It was now out of my hands. I had done everything possible: laid out the severity of the situation, discussed the pregnancy options available (this, a euphemism for pregnancy termination). I did not sway her one way or another. It was non-directive counselling at its best.

Seated at the nursing station, I wondered what I should write in my consultation note. Likely lethal? Probably lethal? Parents appear not to understand the severity of the situation? Counselling ineffective? My chart note reflects none of my despair: "The finding of limb shortening at this early stage of pregnancy may be a significant, if not lethal, skeletal dysplasia"; and "The issue of pregnancy termination may be discussed if the measurements are significantly behind the gestational age." My notes reflect none of the discussions I'd had with Marlene and with Pat Mohide about the severity of the findings; about the shortness of the limbs, the smallness of the chest. Nothing about how awful this child's life might be or how distraught I was by the parents' decision. The fact that my note said that pregnancy termination could "be discussed" later was significant, however; usually, once parents tell me that this is not an option, I document it and do not bring it up again.

At Shannon's appointment three weeks later, the baby's bones had not grown at all. This time, Shannon's father came, too. He squeezed my hand in both of his and shook it with a wide smile on his face.

"Thank you so much, Doctor, for your support," he said. "Shannon said that you're the only one who offered any hope. That you did not give up on the baby."

"We don't know," I said, my brain reeling. What had Shannon told him? "It doesn't look like any skeletal dysplasia I know and we can't predict how severe it'll be."

"Exactly! It may not be so bad after all," he said. "Savannah Rose – that's what they've named her – may be okay."

Oh, no. "I really don't think that she'll be okay," I said. "Her ribs are too short, her lungs will be too small, her bones haven't grown at all in three weeks."

"What will be, will be," Shannon's father said, and Shannon nodded fiercely.

Savannah did need a breathing tube in her throat and a ventilator beside her bassinet from the moment she emerged from the womb. Her minuscule lungs needed all the help they could get to stay inflated. She remained in a neonatal intensive care unit for three months before being transferred to the pediatric one where she stayed long enough to celebrate her first birthday. There, she frequently turned so blue, almost navy blue, from lack of oxygen that the nurses started to call them "Savannah's black spells." Everybody worried about the brain damage they might be causing. She went home – on a ventilator pumping oxygen through a tracheostomy, a surgically created opening in her neck – a month after her first birthday.

During the year that Savannah stayed in the hospital, I was pregnant with Luke. I felt self-conscious from the moment my bump became large enough not to be dismissed as overweight. I was almost ashamed. I worried what it might make my prenatal patients think. Did they envy me for my apparently healthy pregnancy? Did they resent me? At the time, I thought that these pregnant women who carried sick or malformed babies would hate me. My bulging belly suggested I would never have to live their torment or make the kinds of terrible decisions they faced. I imagined them thinking all those things when my belly preceded me into the counselling room, but, really, they were likely so absorbed in their own terrible realities that they probably didn't notice my pregnancy, and if they did, they probably didn't have any emotional reserve to care. Many years later, I received an email from a woman whose name I did not recognize at first. When I opened its attachment, I saw, grinning at me, a boy of African ancestry with an artificial leg and wearing a War Amps T-shirt.

> Dear Dr. Nowaczyk. I am sending you the photo of my son Andre whom you saw in prenatal genetics. You were so wonderful in reassuring us that everything was going to be all right, that he was going to be normal apart from that missing femur that we went home relieved and were able to enjoy the rest of the pregnancy. You were pregnant then, too, and I wondered how could you be doing that job, how difficult it must have been for you. Thank you for your help.

I remembered then: her baby boy had focal femoral deficiency, a partial absence of the thighbone. I had counselled the parents that he would not be intellectually disabled but that the affected leg would likely need to be amputated.

I couldn't believe that a mother faced with such a serious anomaly in her unborn baby would have had the heart to think about another woman's pregnancy, especially if that other woman had just announced that her son would have a serious physical disability. To even notice and acknowledge my pregnancy ... Her generosity stunned me – I'm not sure that I would have been capable of such kindness under similar circumstances.

Two summers after I received that email, during one of Luke's little league baseball games, a boy hop-limped to steal home on his prosthetic left leg. We were playing a team from across town. As his teammates cheered him on wildly when he slid home, I recognized the boy from the photo.

After the game, I crossed the field and asked his father whether during the pregnancy they had seen a prenatal geneticist.

He rose from his lawn chair as I approached. "We saw you," he said and smiled.

"Andre's mom sent me the most lovely letter," I said. "I wouldn't have bothered you otherwise."

"Jeannette isn't here, but she'll be so happy to hear that we saw you."

Jeannette – a warm, African Canadian woman with cornrows and long braids of greying hair – attended the next game our sons played. She enveloped me in her arms.

"You made such a difference," she said and wiped her eyes. "See, I'm still crying."

I did not cry, but I really wanted to.

"Thank you for that email," I said. "You're the only patient who recognized how hard it was for me at the time."

We hugged goodbye. "Thanks for coming over," she said.

I have always loved being a geneticist. Apart from the clinical interactions and the intellectual challenge of chasing zebras, I also loved constantly learning new things. Going to conferences and learning from colleagues before they published their findings, discovering connections between patients and disease processes, delineating new conditions, presenting my unsolved cases – everybody having come with the goal of understanding genetics and advancing knowledge. Interacting with like-minded people just as obsessed and besotted with genetics and sharing stories of the worst cases we have seen – there was solace in this. Of all the physicians in the world, these were the only ones that really understood what it meant to tell an expectant mother that their child was going to have an intellectual disability or that her happily babbling toddler was going to die. Even if I didn't talk much about myself and the toll it was taking on me, I still ended up reassured.

When I began my genetic career, the Human Genome Project – the determination of the entire sequence of human DNA – was about to be completed. The first full sequence of a human chromosome – understandably the second shortest, number 22 (the shortest, 21, actually has more coding sequences than 21) – was published in 1999. Over my twenty-five years of practice, I have seen it result in diagnosis for many patients, finally giving them answers. But we are still far away from providing cures, even for postnatal conditions such as cystic fibrosis (one of the first genes to be identified), despite a biochemistry tutor gushing about its prospects and the "cure being just around the corner" in my first year of medical school back in 1985. Knowing the gene whose mutations cause a disease allows us to understand the disease mechanism better, but many of those genes regulate development and act during embryogenesis; once a child is born the damage is done – the brain connections poorly hooked, the heart valves misaligned, the lip cleft or foot foreshortened. Understanding genes for those sorts of issues is just that – an understanding. The knowledge of which gene caused the defect cannot help to undo the processes. For some functional genes – those that work in postnatal life – understanding the mechanisms of disease is beginning to help in the medical management of some conditions; those are genes for kidney function, hearth rhythm disturbances and certain types of seizures to name a few. But even there, we cannot cure.

My career as a clinical geneticist has been a constant application of new testing technologies. When I began, we only offered karyotyping – the photographic analysis of the number and structure of the chromosomes; several more detailed chromosomal tests that looked for small missing fragments; and sequencing of a handful of genes. Over the past three decades, that number increased exponentially, but the greatest diagnostic game changer has been whole exome sequencing: the simultaneous reading of the sequences of all the gene fragments that code for the building proteins and the enzymes that make the body function. For it to become reality, several scientific developments had to come together: knowing the correct sequence of the genes provided by the Human Genome Project, super-computing power able to handle the terabytes of data generated for each patient, bioinformatics capabilities to sort through it all, and human experience in recognizing and assigning the DNA changes to the physical and functional differences observed in patients. I have sat in several sessions where physicians, researchers, genetic counsellors and a bioinformatician discussed for hours the sequence changes identified by the computing programs that might or might not be responsible for a patient's disease. After all that brute-strength sequencing, after all the data crunching, it was still up to us to make the final call. These discussions are the final step before a gene variant can be assigned as benign or disease-causing.

When it works, it works very well: Tanner, a twenty-year-old man with severe developmental delay whom I have followed in the clinic since he was an infant, was finally diagnosed with Wiedemann-Steiner syndrome after exome sequencing. Until then, I had investigated him with each new test as they became available over the years, but I hadn't seen him for over a decade. "I didn't think you were still working on it," Dayna, his mother, said when I phoned her to tell her about exome sequencing. I was – Tanner was one of the first patients I had seen at McMaster and I thought about him often. When the answer arrived, it was bittersweet: his condition arose as a new mutation and his parents weren't carriers. "I wish I had known about it sooner," Dayna said, "we would have had another baby."

And Warren – the boy with too many fingers and toes. Whole exome sequencing showed that he had a variant of a ciliopathy, confirming the clinical diagnosis of acrocallosal syndrome I had made twenty-one years earlier.

But there are still many patients that do not have a diagnosis – many that I have followed for years. The hope is that once we can sequence all of their DNA (the genome), not only the coding fragments but also the structural and intervening sequences, we will identify their conditions. That, too, is coming. Genetics and I have both come a long way.

☞

When I found myself writing about Savannah in that first creative writing course, at first, I cared only about the truth of my *images* – I wanted my words to show what she looked like to me at that time, I wanted to communicate the suffering I believed she was feeling and how responsible I felt. I cared only about the correspondence of my words to reality, to *my* reality, and I worked painstakingly to select and arrange words to capture that feeling. I know now that my descriptions of Savannah were coloured by my emotions and the inherent judgments of my worldview, and had I been more accepting of her, I would not have used these phrases, these words, to describe her.

In class, I read what I had written:

> I saw her today. Yet another of my professional successes. A fifteen-pound grotesque of foreshortened limbs, crooked vertebrae and blown up skull. Not a single straight bone in her eight-year-old body. I have known her since before she was born, when the grey and black images coalesced to reveal a malformed spine, bowed arms and legs and bent ribs. My many attempts to paint a realistic and warning picture fell on deaf ears; her parents actually tell all that I am the only doctor who never gave up on her.
>
> Now, after almost a year in intensive care units, after many times spend in the hospital with a breathing tube and on ventilator support – her chest and lungs are too small, you see, she is still receiving oxygen by a hole in her throat. Her mother tells me that she is learning to speak in sentences – very short ones because of the breathing problems, and she is learning to use a motorized wheelchair. She loves her eighteen-month-old brother Jack who is already bigger than she is. With squinty little eyes with cataracts and crooked yellowed teeth she looks like a miserable little gargoyle.
>
> What have I done?

The silence in the room after I finished reading still rings in my ears. My classmates sat in silence until one woman burst out: "I hate this. I hate you for making me hear it. How can you be so cruel, describing a helpless, innocent child that way? Have you no heart?"

The teacher didn't comment on my content except to say that she liked "all the 'b' sounds" in it and to comment that the writing was "strong." She then smoothed the ruffled feathers of the upset woman. It was only much later that I wondered how many more in that class had been horrified but chose not to utter a word.

During a break that followed, two women spoke to me in the washroom.

"That woman should not have attacked you," one of them said. "This is supposed to be a safe space for sharing" – a phrase I would later hear repeatedly in many non-professional writing workshops.

"You are so brave to share it with us," said the other.

But I felt like I had accomplished something – my writing had communicated my vision, had elicited a strong response, and that moment of being heard, that lightning possibility of connection through words was all that mattered to me at the time. I didn't realize then that everybody in the class heard my story differently depending on their life histories, their age, their race, their profession – in effect, twenty different versions of Savannah were created by my listeners. Now, I believe I deserved the reaction I got from that woman. It was, perhaps, a punishment for my arrogance, my exuberance, my inexperience; it was perhaps a reminder – like Savannah's life – of the breadth of the human condition.

Would I change what I wrote then knowing what I know now? At the time, my words were accurate – that was how I saw Savannah. Her appearance wasn't pleasing, her voice was raspy and broken up, and – as per aesthetics of the human form – she was ugly. I knew that to her parents Savannah was beautiful, but at the time, I hadn't learned enough to see beyond her physical form. I thought she was suffering, I thought she was unhappy, and in that piece of writing I poured out my horror, including the pain I felt because I had somehow failed this little person, condemned her to a life of discomfort and sorrow.

Was I not allowed to have feelings? I had kept them secret and hidden for so long, and – untold – they festered and hurt me. Maybe I should have shared my feelings with somebody earlier, so that my emotions didn't affect my relationship with Savannah and her parents. I thought I was living up to my profession in supressing my feelings, but they affected the way I saw her.

☞

In spite of all the advances in genetics, I was never able to diagnose Savannah's condition. Over the years, I consulted specialists in skeletal dysplasias from Lausanne, Switzerland, and at the Cedars-Sinai Skeletal Dysplasia Registry in Los Angeles and they were all as stumped as I was. As she grew, I ordered more X-rays and any new genetic test that became available and that I thought might shed some light. I followed her every two years in my clinic. She grew and she learned to walk with a walker over short distances. But all I could see in my clinic was a child who suffered in her body. What I saw as her life and my culpability for it broke my heart every time I saw her and each visit upset me for hours. When she was six, I arranged for whole exome sequencing when it was still a brand-new test in the research stages. Dr. Denny Porter, a researcher at the National Institutes of Health in Bethesda and a friend from the Smith-Lemli-Opitz meetings, agreed to do it free of charge, but Shannon and Shane did not come in for the necessary blood tests. Their DNA samples were needed to compare with Savannah's. Without them the testing could not proceed. They did not reschedule their appointment and I was a bit miffed. Did they not want to know the cause of their daughter's condition? I know I did. But I also recognized that they were telling me something and I did not pursue the issue further.

I stayed miserable about her for years. I couldn't see how wonderful she was and how happy. I hid my pain behind the search for a diagnosis and pretended that everything was all right.

☞

But being a good geneticist and a good doctor was not all about the hunt for zebras.

One day in my clinic, Justin, fifteen, unable to walk or talk and still in diapers, flopped in his custom-form wheelchair; his thin limbs pretzelled onto themselves in his stroller. We hadn't determined if he could see but we knew that he was deaf; his face lacked any expression. At conferences where I had presented his case, other geneticists were as stumped as I was: he did not have a recognizable syndrome. All his genetic tests had come back as normal. At this appointment, I wanted to discuss with his mother a panel of next-generation sequencing that might identify a genetic mutation and finally find a diagnosis.

But as I searched for new clues on Justin's physical examination, a long-held suspicion coalesced into a truth in my mind: with time, for some patients and for some parents, naming the disease simply did not matter. Justin was Justin. No point in poking him for more blood or spinal fluid, putting a bag over his penis to collect urine or sedating him for another MRI. His mother agreed, relief audible in her voice. She did not want her son to be treated like an interesting specimen anymore; a diagnosis would not change anything for her or for him. And since she and her husband did not plan to have any more children, there was no longer the pressing need to identify the cause, at least not until his sister began to consider having children herself.

At this moment in her life, Justin's mother simply wanted to talk. So, I sat and listened to her. And, from that day forward, to many other parents.

Of course, I continued to search for diagnoses for other patients – for prenatal cases, for newborns with unexpected anomalies, for children with intellectual disability. I counselled parents who wanted to have more children and patients' siblings who were starting their own families. But for many patients and their parents, being heard was just as, if not more, important.

13.

The May after I returned from Homewood, I flew to Warsaw for a book tour for my second book. I'd finished writing *Family Tree of Health* after my discharge from the hospital. My publisher had been so pleased with the success of *Searching for Ancestors* that he requested a companion volume on genetics. On the afternoon of the launch, as I walked along a sun-drenched street, birds chirping in the spring-green trees, elegant Europeans daintily drinking espresso in street cafés, Jimm phoned and informed me that Jack had been suspended from school because he'd "hit a teacher."

Jimm had just come from a meeting where Jack's homeroom teacher, his gym teacher and the middle school principal had ambushed him. It was painfully obvious to Jimm that none of them wanted Jack in their fancy-schmancy school. Jimm talked and talked, agitated, distraught, as I rushed toward the baroque Staszic Palace in the centre of Warsaw. There, a popular Polish TV personality was going to introduce me, and a genealogist who had worked on the Polish edition of the BBC's *Who Do You Think You Are?*, a program where celebrities searched for their ancestors, was going to interview me.

I could not calm Jimm down. I had to hang up on him mid-sentence as I stepped across the wide oak threshold of the palace. My hands shook as I climbed the wide marble stairs and entered a room full of people, but somehow, I managed to deliver – the photos from the launch show me smiling next to the celebrities. My insides, though, were roiling. What was the point of writing books when my personal life was in shambles? Who cared about a genetics book when my family was falling apart?

☞

Two days later, the arrivals doors at Pearson International Airport whooshed open on Jack, who stood there sad and terrified behind the arrivals glass bannister. All alone, apart from Jimm and Luke, he searched my face with his big blue eyes. Such a lost, small little guy with such huge anguish on his thin shoulders. I hugged him so hard, his ribs dug into my breasts as his skinny arms hung limp beside his body – he had never been a hugger. I said, "Oh, Jack," over and over, reduced to my monosyllabic misery yet again.

We took him out of that private school. The principal had demanded that Jack undergo another battery of psychological tests and hinted at using medication. The incident, "hitting a teacher," turned out to be nothing more than Jack pushing aside a teacher's arm when he blocked his exit as the kids thronged to leave. When, in solidarity, we took Luke out of the school as well, the principal announced that we owed the school Luke's tuition for the year as it was too late in the summer for them to fill his spot. Jimm wrote a terse yet eloquent reply telling them what he thought about it.

In September, we enrolled Jack in the local middle school and I met his new homeroom teacher – a stocky, tattooed man with a no-crap manner – two weeks after the school year started. He had reviewed Jack's file and he told me that it reminded him of similar files belonging to kids who did not finish high school. Oh, okay, I thought, Jack won't finish high school. The significance of his statement did not register at all until that evening when Jimm said angrily, "So he'll be a high school dropout?" Somehow, I made peace with that – therapy and all the work I'd done at Homewood in action. But Jack did well in middle school. He made friends, he played hockey, he behaved. His learning disability led to easy frustration and – like in his mother – quick anger, but he managed with those, too. After he graduated from middle school, he went to Westdale Secondary School, the local high school that also happened to boast the highest academic standards in Hamilton. There, he thrived: he made friends without difficulty; he played football. He studied hard and received academic honours. He needed tutors for math and physics, but in humanities and social sciences he got As throughout. Before he graduated grade twelve in 2014, he had received scholarships to four Ontario universities. He chose Queen's University in Kingston and graduated with a BA in political science four years later, followed by a law degree from the University of Southampton Law School. While I was editing this memoir, he finished a Master of Laws degree at Osgoode Hall Law School in Toronto.

☞

Our little family hobbled along. In August 2007, at the age of fifty-six, Jimm's older brother, Kosta, was diagnosed with pancreatic cancer and barely survived the surgery to remove the tumour. For the next twelve months, the leaden cloud of his illness darkened our life. He died almost exactly a year after his surgery. Jimm was devastated – Kosta was the last of his immediate family that he had lost to cancer.

The following year, on a mid-April evening still cool with lingering winter, my mother phoned me around 9:30 p.m.

"I came back from work and found Tato lying on the floor in the kitchen," she said, her voice shot with panic. "He can't get up. He's talking nonsense."

She passed the receiver to my father and I heard a moan. On some level his moans seemed to make sense – their intonation varied as I asked him questions but maybe I only imagined it. When my mother took the receiver back, I told her to call an ambulance. Our next-door neighbour stayed with Jack and Luke, and, barrelling up Highway 407, Jimm and I arrived at the Milton District Hospital before the ambulance carrying my father pulled into the emergency bay. When the paramedics opened the rear door and lifted out the stretcher, I rushed to my father's side and told him I was there, that everything would be all right.

"Ma'am, he's unconscious," the paramedic said.

"But I just spoke with him!" And with dismay I realized that I had not told him that I loved him before my mother took the receiver from him. The regret gnaws at me to this day.

☞

My father never regained consciousness. He must have hit his head when he fell: the CT scan showed a massive hemorrhage that filled the left side of his brain. Because his alcohol-destroyed liver did not produce clotting factors, the bleeding continued, and by the afternoon of the next day the doctors could no longer continue life support; all the blood transfused into his veins to maintain his blood pressure pooled in his brain and compressed the breathing centre in his brainstem. Even machines couldn't keep his body alive. My father's brain – his intelligence, his personality, his kindness, his generosity – were gone. He was gone.

For several hours, I couldn't reach Monika in Cambodia. Finally, I called my brother-in-law: they were on a cruise on the Mekong River and Monika's cell had ran out of battery. Even if Monika could get on the next flight to Toronto from Hong Kong or Bangkok, she would not arrive for at least thirty-six hours.

Later, Monika told me about a dream she'd had the night she returned to Phnom Penh, just before she left for the airport to catch the flight to Toronto. "Tato was standing by the door to my room with that smile of his, just looking at me." I knew that smile: head tilted slightly to the left, wide-stretched but closed lips, kind and loving eyes. My sister continued, "'See,' I said to him, 'I knew you'd be all right.'"

He wasn't. Soon, I had to call her again to tell her that we were turning off the life supports even before she could leave Phnom Penh. "We can't keep him alive until you come back," I explained as we both sobbed into the phone. She said she understood.

"You're so stupid!" I shouted at my father when the ICU physician switched off his respirator later that afternoon. I grabbed his hand and shook it. "You promised!" He had promised me that he would be there when Jack graduated from university because he had believed so strongly in my son's abilities. I needed my father to be alive to keep the faith. "You're just so stupid!" I was livid because he had not stopped drinking, because he didn't care enough about himself or about us. He could have lived much, much longer if he had quit.

Jimm peeled my fingers from my father's hand, one by one. He hugged me and I finally cried.

The intensive care unit was on the second storey of the hospital. A curtained window facing south spanned the wall. I twisted out of Jimm's arms and walked around my father's bed. I swept the bile-yellow curtains aside and light flooded the room, motes of dust dancing on the sunrays. Beyond the window stretched the dingy April fields of Southern Ontario, barren brush and skeletal trees scratching at the horizon. The pale sun past its zenith sailed toward the west. The view reminded me of the field behind my father's childhood home in Lasek, where he had roamed as a boy, chasing and being chased by his mother's hissing geese. I remembered the orchard where he had climbed the apple trees for that mouth-puckering first bite of the season; where starlings and crows swirled in a cloud above his head; where his mother's voice called him and his sisters home for the simple dinner she had prepared. I wanted his soul to fly there, into the happiness of his childhood.

I turned to my father and held his hand.

"Go," I said. "Go run in the fields again. They're waiting for you."

A week after my father's funeral, the phrase "narrative medicine" caught my eye on a flyer pasted to the wall between two elevators on the second floor of McMaster Children's Hospital. It was an announcement for the annual Henry and Sylvia Wong Forum in Medicine, a lecture titled "A Health Care Transformed by Stories." Intrigued, I read on:

> Narrative Medicine is a clinical practice fortified by the knowledge of what to do with stories. A child gets leukaemia, a senior breaks her hip, an adolescent girl gets pregnant, a grandmother loses her mind, a young mother finds a breast lump, an infant is born with a damaged heart. We, clinicians, enter these complex narrative situations having to imagine what the situation must be like from the inside and having to imagine alternative futures for these patients and their families. We are learning about powerful methods that increase the narrative competence of all healthcare

professionals, enabling them to honour their patients' stories of illness and to provide singular and effective health care. As a dividend, narrative medicine also nourishes individual health care professionals and strengthens the team-work upon which we always rely.

I had no idea what much of it meant, but narrative medicine seemed to combine two things dear to me: literature and the practice of medicine. It resonated with my lifelong love of reading literature and poetry, and with my desire to write, to communicate my experiences through words. I thought narrative medicine had something to do with telling stories of medicine, something I had always wanted to do. Curiosity brought me to the lecture hall the following week to experience, for the first time, Dr. Rita Charon enchanting an audience with a vision of what the practice of medicine could be when combined with a narrative approach.

"Narrative medicine is a medical approach that utilizes people's narratives in clinical practice, research, and education as a way to promote healing," reads the Wikipedia entry. Rita's definition is more eloquent and elegant: narrative medicine is the "ability to recognize, absorb, interpret and act on the stories and plights of others."

But what exactly does either of these two definitions mean?

Misconceptions about narrative medicine abound. Most people – like I did – think it has to do with physicians telling patients' stories. Some joke that "narrative medicine" is a narrative prescribed to the patient like "cough medicine," a piece of writing given in a dose to provide a health benefit. Instead, the practice is a means of improving the listening skills of doctors with the ultimate aim of accurate diagnosis and improved medical management.

The narrative medicine movement arose in the late twentieth century in reaction to the increasing technologization and dehumanization of clinical medicine, independently in the United States and in England. In the tangle of leads and sensors and machines documenting the patient's every breath, heartbeat or brainwave, physicians were rapidly forgetting the person at the centre. In 1999, I witnessed it firsthand when a medical student told me that he did not need to learn how to take a baby's pulse because the monitor over her bassinet displayed it continuously. My jaw dropped, literally. I asked him what he planned to specialize in. His answer – "adult cardiology" – did not surprise me at all; cardiologists had long before stopped taking hold of patient's wrists to count their heartbeat, relying instead on increasingly complex and sophisticated machines and sensors to evaluate the rhythms of people's hearts. They were more likely to explore the inside of the patient's heart in the angiography suite when squirting radioopaque dye into her coronary vessels than to lay a hand on her chest to feel the drum of the heart.

Somewhere in that technological maze people got lost; the stories of their lives and illnesses were buried under printouts of their blood test results, long tracings of their pulse and blood pressure, breathing patterns and brainwaves. As doctors, we were reaching deeper and deeper into human bodies, but we were leaving behind the people inhabiting those bodies. We weren't listening to them. Narrative medicine attempted to bring the patient's story to the forefront again; to place a patient's experience alongside technology as being equally important.

Rita Charon received her medical degree from Harvard Medical School in 1978 and trained in internal medicine at Montefiore Hospital in New York City. She studied English literature and defended her PhD thesis in 1999 at Columbia University's Department of English and Comparative Literature.

The way Rita tells the story, after several years of practicing internal medicine, she realized that what patients paid her to do was to listen to complicated narratives told in words, gestures, silences, tracings, images, blood tests and physical findings, and to cohere all these into something that made enough sense to act on. As the patient told his or her own – sometimes very difficult – story, the job of the physician was to "hear" it competently and attentively. Rita's brilliance led her to realize that the specialists in the telling and understanding of stories lived in the departments of English literature, where she hastened for instruction. Her first English literature course morphed into master's-level courses and, soon after that, a doctoral degree in English literature.

Rita discovered that the study of literature made her a better doctor by making her a better "reader" of what her patients were saying. She learned that the same attention required for an in-depth study of literary texts (called close reading) could be harnessed to improve the listening skills of health-care professionals. By paying close attention to the "text" of the patient, a listening physician can garner a lot more information than what is conveyed by the bare meaning of the words: the patient's word choices, her silences and omissions, her metaphors and figures of speech all provide additional information and data. Eventually, Rita and others made the study of narrative part of the Columbia medical school curriculum. A few years later, they established a Master of Science program in Narrative Medicine, but not before she had been dubbed Columbia University's "crazy book lady."

During the Wong Forum at McMaster, Rita invited us to experience what it means to tell a story and to hear a story written by another. She asked us to write for five minutes and then to share what we wrote with our neighbour to the right. I don't remember the prompt – Rita always uses prompts for writing – but I do remember that I wrote about my father's death. I missed him terribly, every day. Still do. The girl to my right listened and told me that her grandmother had also died recently and that my writing reminded her of her.

Rita's lecture, while delivered with her breathless attention and piercing stare, earnest and eloquent, did not yield an epiphany. But something in her demeanour – her utter conviction that her approach was worthwhile and important – something in that birdlike, impassioned woman resonated within me. Something told me that I should listen to her some more. A year later, in October 2010, I flew to New York City for Columbia University's introductory narrative medicine weekend workshop.

On the Friday afternoon, Rita welcomed us in the classroom on the third floor of the Hamilton Hall on the Columbia campus as if we were her long-lost prodigal children. She told us about *Volvox*, a strain of green algae that had, over a relatively short period of time of thirty-five million years – more than two hundred million years ago – developed an ability to form self-contained colonies with a division of labour between cells, essentially modelling the evolution of multicellular organisms. She compared our group of health-care professionals interested in practicing narrative medicine to a *Volvox* colony. She described how the first single-celled organisms did everything themselves – grow, propel across the waters they lived in, reproduce – and how, in the colony, some gave up the ability to reproduce and began to secrete the goo that surrounded the colony; others used their cilia to enact movement, and others still specialized in reproduction. She told us that we, too, were learning to rely on each other. That we were becoming a colony with a single unifying purpose.

Rita has this wonderful way of connecting biological processes with the collaborative process of narrative medicine. In her paper "At the Membranes of Care," she compared communication between people across what she describes as the "membranes of ignorance" to the action of biological ligands. These molecules bind to cellular membranes and effect changes inside the cell just like powerful stories change our perceptions and our consciousness, and bind us together in the experience of being human. Her work in narrative medicine consists of teaching physicians the tools of close reading to improve their listening skills, and the practices of reflective and creative writing to encourage introspection. In learning the skill of close reading, students parse the frame, form, timeline, plot and desire of the literary story, all of which can then be applied, almost instinctively, in the outpatient clinic, on the ward or in the emergency room, to get at the crux of a patient's experience. This careful attention not only validates the personal history of the patient but also encourages self-reflection in the physician.

Reflective writing by physicians articulates the emotional underpinnings of both their patients' stories and their own. When writing about an encounter after it has occurred, a doctor has the luxury of time and distance to evaluate his or her reactions and emotions, and to determine if and how those might have affected the diagnostic process. During reflective writing, for example, a physician might name his or her feelings toward a patient or refer to a patient as "difficult" or "an unreliable historian."

Labels like this are certain to affect information gathering and perhaps even the arc of a patient's care, but the writing enables the physician to move beyond themselves, to understand why they perceived the patient as such.

During the weekend-long workshop, we experienced the three arms of narrative medicine – close listening, reflective writing and parallel charting – in several practice sessions. Instead of charting on patients in medicalese – coded medical language that allows no room for physician or patient feelings – we were encouraged to document patient encounters in plain English. The "parallel chart," Rita's invention, houses writing about the deeply emotional parts of being a doctor and allows doctors to reflect on patient care from a holistic stance. Lectures on narrative ethics, empathy and creative writing completed the whole.

At the workshops, we were divided up into small groups in which we would spend the weekend. Along with our facilitator for the first session, Nellie Hermann, a critically acclaimed novelist and the Creative Director of the Narrative Medicine Program, eight students – seven women and one man – sat around a cracked faux pine-topped table. We cast sidelong glances at one another, nervous and uncertain as to what to expect. Nellie quickly explained the rules. For the duration of the weekend, the workshop was a safe place with confidentiality as key – nothing was to be repeated or discussed outside the room.[4] We did not have to participate in the writing if we did not want to and we could pass on reading aloud what we wrote. We could leave at any time without explanation.

"When it's your turn to read, do it without a preamble and read exactly what you wrote," Nellie said. Then she asked us to "write the story of our name."

"First or last?" somebody asked.

"Whichever you choose."

---

4   I have obtained permission from Rita Charon as well as all the classmates identified by name to share our experiences here.

As I wrote on my usual letter-size, yellow paper pad, I was surprised that Nellie was writing as well. I wondered how many times she had done this before.

I wrote:

> I am one of the twice-named, as per Robertson Davies. I was christened Małgorzata when I was three days old, but by the time I turned eighteen I changed it to Margaret. Essentially the same name, but what a divide – Margaret is solid, immutable, ever-so-English, while in Polish the name changes according to who calls you. It can mean so many things. And with a new name, I forged myself as the successful, achieving, excelling physician. And I did not go back to the old name for twenty-three years. I have now reclaimed it somewhat, and friends in Poland call me – whatever [names] they choose are appropriate. And it helped me (?), informs me re: what they think about me. But Margaret is always the same (or supposed to be, my husband calls me that and he wished me to be a certain way). Cast in stone, solid, reliable, dependable, immutable. But my Polish names are like my moods and feelings and craziness and other stuff. So I molded myself in this name and by now I have been Margaret twice as long as I have been ...

And Nellie said, "Finish this last sentence."

We went around the table to read. Katherine read how much she had disliked her given name, disliked it until she married a man of French-Canadian ancestry and finally liked its pairing with his Québécois surname. Krisann wrote that she had thought that her name came from "chrysanthemum," Nadia that she had been named after a prima ballerina with whom her mother studied ballet in England. After I read my notes, Thomas said that now he understood why his Polish grandmother had different names for him when he was little. "I never liked it. It was confusing that she had all those names for me," he said. The ice had been broken and we were ready for the rest of the weekend.

☞

The following morning, we met with a different facilitator to discuss Dostoyevsky's story "A Gentle Creature," in which a young woman has committed suicide by jumping from a window, clutching a religious icon. Her husband, who arrives at the scene moments after her death, struggles to understand her act. His attempts to tell the story of their life together can be viewed as attempts to comprehend, to move on, to heal after the trauma. Yet as he rambles on, her motives elude him, although they become increasingly clear to the reader – he had been a tyrannical husband who manipulated and controlled her even before their marriage. He tells his story in fits and starts, and persists in justifying his behaviour toward her, finally arriving at self-forgiveness and self-pity, now a loving husband in his mind – a conversion that he believes had been denied to him by her suicide.

The story is narratively complex: the timeline is not linear – it loops back into the past only to jump forward into the future; the diction is archaic, complex and confusing, not least because the narrator is intent on showing himself in the best possible light. The characters remain unnamed for a long time. The woman's voice is mediated through the husband's telling of her story and it soon becomes obvious that the narrator is not only unreliable and incomprehensible but also despicable.

For us as doctors and health-care practitioners, Dostoyevsky's narrator was the embodiment of both the "hateful patient" and the "unreliable historian." By the end of the session, however, having parsed the story in literary terms, we reached the point that we could if not understand his motives at least have a better sense of him as a person. This exercise was a practical demonstration of how close reading of a literary text fosters empathy. And while it was quite obvious from our first reading of the story why the narrator's wife had jumped – because she was married to an odious control freak with mutable morals – we continued to argue about the narrator's impulses and deeds, epiphanies and breakthroughs. The net effect, as simplistic as it sounds, was the beginning of an understanding toward the unpleasant narrator and, by extension, of the moral complexities and life stories of people we deal with in medical practice.

☞

During the "Narrative Writing from Practice" session on Saturday afternoon, the time came to share the writing that we had been asked to bring to the workshop – a story about a clinical encounter that we felt we could, and wanted to, read to others. I had not realized until that moment that the chance to read my writing was what had brought me to New York City.

Rita happened to be the facilitator assigned to this session, and as she explained the purpose of that workshop, I felt fear coursing through my arteries and veins. My heart was pounding. I had brought my piece about Savannah that I had written and read to my creative writing class with such disastrous consequences. I felt the time had come to finally discuss the effect the story had had on me as a physician and as a person.

I panicked. I'm not chickening out at the last minute, I thought. I must get something out of this whole trip. I will forever regret it if I don't volunteer. My hand shot up. Rita glanced at me and nodded, and I began reading.

☞

Sunday morning, the roster assigned Rita to our small group for the afternoon session, "Bearing Witness to the Suffering of Others." Taking turns, we read Sharon Olds's poem "The Death of Marilyn Monroe," and then Rita prompted us to "write about the suffering of someone who moved you."

I choked. I had no idea who to write about. I began with "Am I totally unfeeling?" and continued:

> Who can I choose – whoever it is it will be about me – my needs, then and now, my point of view. I want to be absolved of that death I caused – she died because I was too tired to wake up, to go in, to see her, to attend to her – I just told the resident to give her Advil. I should have known that I needed to see her, examine her, dialyze her that night. Don and others have kept her alive for twelve years and here I killed her. Because Jack wasn't sleeping through the night, because I can't function on three hours of sleep, because I

was not awake when they called me.

Next day she was comatose and in ICU. No dialysis, no supports would change the outcome. She lingered with a severely swollen brain for a couple of days until the decision was made to withdraw.

And as she lay there dying, in a room full of people I was offered a place of honour by parents at the head of her bed. When her breathing stopped, her parents hugged me.

I saw them walking hand in hand along the street later that afternoon, my husband was driving me home, and offering me solace and support for I was just through.

I attended her funeral two days later. Four of us drove 80 km away …

And I heard Rita say, "Finish this last sentence."

Again, I had that feeling: "I'm going to do it." I was ready to burst, to spill open; if I did not share, I would regret it for the rest of my life. I think I might have ruptured an artery in my brain had I not lifted my hand.

So again, I read out loud my misery and my shame.

☞

"What did you hear?" Rita asked the silence.

"How guilty she feels," Krisann said.

"The remorse. The sorrow," Cheryl said, and smiled at me across the table.

"She was tired – the fatigue," Thomas said. "I can still hear it in her words now."

"Yes, what was that? Can you read it again?" Rita asked me.

"'Because Jack wasn't sleeping through the night, because I can't function on three hours of sleep, because I was not awake when they called me.'"

"Yes, that," Rita said.

"I was on call. I should've gone in," I said.

"You were exhausted," Rita said. "Show some compassion."

Compassion? For myself? I was not brought up that way; that was not how I'd functioned during my career. Would things have been different had I gone to the hospital in the middle of the night? Maybe this had been Clara's night to die no matter what I did. Maybe even if I had examined her at three in the morning, she would still have slipped into a coma, never to wake. What if I had put her on dialysis that night? Maybe she wouldn't have deteriorated so fast. Had I gone in, I would have had the clear conscience of having done everything I could, but I didn't. The mistakes of omission haunt us the most. If you do everything you can and make a mistake, it might be acceptable. But to not do everything is an unforgivable offence, my conscience was telling me.

Again, I had shown the worst side of myself in a roomful of health-care workers and still they accepted me as a human being. Rita and the group were telling me to forgive myself, to treat myself with kindness and to take care of myself. It made the whole weekend worthwhile. Impulsively, I asked Rita if she would be my adopted aunt, and she – with a twinkle in her eye – said yes, she would.

☞

Sitting in the Buffalo airport that evening waiting for the hired car to take me back to Hamilton, I wrote frantic notes from those three days. I could have flown home without the airplane, I felt so unweighted. All the feelings, all the emotions I had held back, closed off, geysered out of me.

The guilt over Clara's death had haunted me for fourteen years, over Savannah's birth for almost ten. I had never shared those stories with anyone other than Jimm but they were not his burdens to bear. These stories ate at my innards, took permanent residence in my memory like pebbles in my shoe that I couldn't shake out.

I balanced my notebook in my lap and wrote and wrote and wrote. I wanted to capture this feeling of lightness. I had found them, finally, people who understood me, accepted me without judgment and respected me.

In the heat of the moment, I did not yet realize that it wasn't only the writing but the sharing, the opening up to others, that had made all the difference to me, in me. I only knew then how light I felt in my body, how much happier, how sane. The receiving of my story, the acceptance of the imperfect me was shocking. It was only the second time in my life that I felt completely accepted with all my flaws and blemishes and uncertainties – the first was with Jimm, when we were dating. I did not have to be perfect. I did not have to hide my doubts and warts. I had always presented an unruffled, devil-may-care attitude. Did I hide because of my fear of rejection? Because I had always been judged so harshly as a child? Or is this too facile an explanation? Whatever the reason, the feeling of wholesale acceptance was transporting.

My notes are a jumble of scribbles, pressured, flattened by speed, as they poured out of me: "I cannot believe how liberating it was. How liberating it feels. I have room in my chest, I have space in my stomach. I did not realize how I carried these two cases with me and how they bore into me, how they became a part of my marrow and of my brain." The new space I found in my chest and in my belly "made room for more." I knew then and there – in the dingy Buffalo International Airport arrivals hall – that I would keep writing.

☞

Two months after my return from New York City, I received a consult on a woman at thirty-three weeks of pregnancy – an ultrasound had detected "an abnormal profile" in her baby girl. In the radiology suite, the baby's ultrasound images showed a bulging forehead, a tiny nubbin of a nose and prominent lips, but the heart, lungs, kidneys and brain all appeared normal. When I entered the counselling room in which the mother had been waiting with her husband, I had no idea what the baby may have.

The woman looked vaguely pugilistic: thick, crimson lips, a broad nose and a wide chin. Her face glowed as if she had sat in the sun for too long. When she said hello, her voice resonated almost as deep as her husband's baritone.

I explained the ultrasound images and admitted that I didn't know what was going on with the baby. "I don't think we'll know until she's born," I said. "You have thick lips, so maybe the baby comes by it honestly." Reassure, I thought, write your notes; deal with the baby when she's born, it's too late to do anything at this late stage of pregnancy.

"This is not the way I normally look," the mother said.

I'd like to think that I would have heeded these words without the training in attentive listening, but "narrative medicine" flashed in my mind at that moment.

"What do you mean?" I asked.

"That's true," her husband said. "She's been telling her doctor and midwife but they keep saying it's just the pregnancy."

This is not the way she looks, I repeated in my mind. Whatever this was supposed to mean, nobody had paid attention to what she had been saying.

"Do you have a photo of yourself from before?" I asked.

Her husband pulled out his phone. Chiselled cheekbones, aquiline nose, skin as clear as porcelain. I looked from the photo to the woman before me and back at the photo, mind whirring as her husband said, "April, just before she got pregnant."

The evidence before me "moved me to action," as Rita would say. After three weeks of blood tests and investigations, we found testosterone levels four times the upper normal limit in the woman's blood; the endocrinologist suspected that she had a tumour either in her ovary or her adrenal gland, a common cause of elevated androgens in a woman. But four weeks later, after the baby girl was born with anomalies of her airway and skeleton – none of which were detectable on ultrasounds – I made the diagnosis of a rare biochemical condition that causes excess production of testosterone in the baby. The testosterone level was so high, it spilled across the placenta into the mother's bloodstream and caused her to become virilized: over several months nobody noticed the changes in this young woman's body because nobody heard what she was saying. I almost made the same mistake when I first saw her.

☞

I did keep my promise to keep writing. After two more creative writing classes with Catherine Graham, I dropped into a chair at my dining room table one August afternoon and, with Jack and Luke playing noisy war games behind and beneath me, a story loosely based on that dreadful ultrasound during my pregnancy with Jack poured out of me. After two rounds of edits with my best writing friend, I submitted "Certainty" to *The Examined Life Journal*, a medical literary journal at the Carver College of Medicine at the University of Iowa, and it was published in 2011. I signed up for online courses at the School of Continuing Studies at the University of Toronto and submitted a story to their Random House–sponsored contest – I ended up a finalist. In 2013, I applied to and was accepted into the Master of Fine Arts in Creative Writing at the University of British Columbia – my writerly dream finally come true. The seeds of this memoir sprouted in a creative non-fiction class I took there in 2016 and became my thesis, which I defended in 2018.

Jimm supported my dreams of becoming a writer from the very beginning. Even before I allowed myself to take it seriously, he found books on writing in the public library and brought them home.

"Why did you get me this?" I would ask, holding *Writer's Gym* or *How to Become a Famous Writer Before You're Dead*, the latter making me suspicious that he was making fun of me.

"I thought you wanted to be a writer," was all he said.

In my quest to learn more about narrative medicine, I read books by Arthur Frank on the patient experience as a story and by Arthur Kleinman on illness narratives. In my reading, I came across a terribly dated book by the anthropologist Charles L. Bosk. *All God's Mistakes* – a horrible, judgmental title – reported on an ethnographic study of clinical geneticists from a Midwestern tertiary hospital, with chapters titled "Genetic Counselling as Dirty Work" and "Mopping-Up," and presented geneticists as callous and brutal truth-tellers – definitely not narrative medicine. Neither was Robert Marion's *Genetic Rounds*. I eagerly waited for it to arrive at my local library because I thought that a book written by a clinical geneticist would illuminate my dilemmas better than a book written by another specialist. What a disappointment: it merely served as a showcase for its author's brilliant diagnostic skills. I threw it across the room after reading one of the more maudlin and self-aggrandizing passages. The author took patients' stories and pain and used them to anoint himself as a super clinician – something Rita and the other faculty had warned against in the lecture on narrative ethics, and throughout the whole workshop.

Wanting to spread knowledge of narrative medicine, in 2012, I published an article on how narrative medicine can be used specifically in clinical genetics and, with the support of Dr. John Carey, editor-in-chief of the *American Journal of Medical Genetics*, launched Frameshifts, a narrative medicine column in the journal. In 2014, I published a paper on narrative medicine for a Polish internal medicine monthly, which was also translated into German. I plugged the benefits of narrative medicine whenever and wherever I could. I gave talks and ran workshops at McMaster and at SickKids.

I became a regular at the Examined Life Conference, hosted by the Carver College of Medicine at the University of Iowa, where every year health-care professionals and patients learned from each other how to use arts in humanizing medicine. I ran a workshop on how to begin and continue writing. In the fall of 2016, I stood in front of the entire conference audience in a dimly lit lecture hall and read "Almost Perfect," a non-fiction piece about the gene that causes Tay-Sachs disease and a little girl I had seen with it as a resident. Jason Lewis, the conference organizer, had asked me to open the conference with *my* writing.

With all this work I was doing, it became clearer and clearer to me that physicians need not be afraid to show their feelings and emotions. The emotional gatekeeping that I had witnessed during my training, the tough persona modelled by the attendings, is not necessary; in fact, it is ill-advised. A few years ago, an ICU physician at McMaster Children's Hospital was in charge of a teenage girl who died as a result of medical error. The girl's father sued the hospital and all the personnel involved. The ICU physician had wanted to speak to the father but had been advised against it by his lawyers, something I remember from my interaction with the Canadian Medical Protective Association. In the past, an investigation – the so-called

Morbidity and Mortality rounds – had only one goal: to identify the root causes of the incident in order to prevent it from happening again. Physicians and residents were crucified at the altar of medical investigation and competency. There was never any thought toward offering support to the medical personnel, nor was there an opportunity for them to express their feelings. This physician recently recalled his journey in the *University of Toronto Medical Journal* in an issue devoted to physician wellness. He'd become depressed and his marriage had fallen apart. I wonder how much of this unhappiness could have been avoided had he been able to speak freely to the girl's father and to his colleagues.

Physicians can show emotions without calling attention to themselves or taking away from their patients' suffering, and in doing so they can retain emotional health and resiliency. Simple tools are available: reading literature to gain insight into human nature that might be different from ours, writing about our emotions in order to process them, and talking with others without shame or guilt, even if we did make a mistake and, especially, if we didn't. Examining and expressing our feelings can only benefit us and, in turn, our patients. Narrative medicine teaches clinicians to see the patient as equal, with all her faults and merits, fully individuated. That was the message that I have carried with me to meetings and conferences, and that has guided me in my clinical practice ever since.

But I still had unfinished business. I followed Rita's prescription of "reframing" Savannah. I talked to the intensive care physician who for years had managed her ventilator needs. I talked to Savannah's G-tube nurse who followed her regularly for surgical site care (making sure that the opening in her abdomen functioned well) and for nutrition. I learned that at school, she ruled a bevy of friends who fought for the privilege of pushing her wheelchair, and that she arbitrated math – she always got the correct answers first. Her younger brother Jack adored her. Everybody agreed: Savannah was happy. Savannah loved her life.

Why didn't I see any of that in my clinic? Had the pursuit of perfection – imbued, drilled into me since childhood – obscured what was right in front of me? Was it the judgment – always harsh – that deflated me after the least of my transgressions? Only perfection deserved praise and acceptance, only unmarred beauty – those were the hard lessons of my childhood that I had to unlearn.

☞

And then one sunny September day in 2013, Savannah complained of a headache. The following morning, she woke up with half of her face and the side of her head swollen and crimson. In the emergency room the next day, a head CT scan showed a brain hemorrhage. Her bones were so soft and yielding that they bulged out under the pressure of the accumulated blood and prevented her from dying instantly, said the neurosurgeon who operated on her.

I visited her in the pediatric intensive care after her surgery, the walls of her room covered with banners, posters and get-well cards. Neon pink–framed sunglasses perched on her face – she looked cheeky, irreverent, even though she was unconscious. Two teachers from her school took turns reading the messages and signatures on the cards they had just delivered. But eventually, the brain swelling caused an irreversible injury to her brainstem and she died three days later.

Her funeral was a party, a celebration, not a scene of mourning. Shannon and Shane had booked two of the largest adjacent rooms in the funeral home and they overflowed with people. Kids ran around playing catch; Savannah's posse giggled in a clutch and pointed to the photos on the walls; adults lined up to speak to Shannon, Shane and Jack who stood in the receiving line. I circled the room, examining the hundreds of photos glued to bristol boards: Savannah at school, Savannah with Jack, Savannah with her grandparents – I recognized her grandfather from that prenatal visit – Savannah on a beach and on a snowy slope bundled into a sled. Always smiling.

Only one photo showed Savannah with a doctor. Savannah in the pediatric ICU on the day she went home. I am propping her for the photo that

Shannon shot, a thick, corrugated bright blue hose connecting the hole in Savannah's throat to a respirator. I am smiling, but I'm sure that I was thinking that this was crazy, inhuman, to let this child suffer so.

I had been so wrong.

But my greatest epiphany happened when I picked up the commemorative leaflet Shannon had printed. On a yellow background scattered with butterflies fluttering above marigolds, above her smiling photo, her full name was printed in bold letters – Savannah Rose.

In my misery and confusion, I had forgotten her beautiful name.

Coda

My first piece of writing poured out of me after my father suffered his heart attack in 1989. Titled "My Father's Heart," I hoped to publish it in a humanities column in a medical journal but it perished in the bowels of our IBM-clone desktop computer sometime in the early 1990s.

I wish I had kept on writing.

With experiences that trouble us, that diminish the space inside of us, writing, by moving the internal to the external, allows us to make room for more – exactly what had happened to me when I shared my two stories in the workshop in New York City. Tying together ideas and experiences across time and place, writing has helped me understand what has happened to me. Writing is a tool to cope and to recover, right at my fingertips. It connects me with others: writers, readers, patients, colleagues. My writing does not let me bullshit myself – even if I start out fake, I end up facing truths that clamour to be let out by my words, my sentences.

As this memoir began to take shape, I realized how big a role reframing and telling my version of Savannah's story had on my mental health recovery. But could I include the details of her life, details that crossed into matters of patient confidentiality, of privacy and ethics? Even if I changed her name, everybody who has worked at McMaster Children's Hospital in the past twenty years would know who she was. And I wanted to keep her name – Savannah Rose. It resonated so beautifully with what Rita had advised. My forgetting the second element underscored how darkly I'd seen Savannah all these years.

Shannon, Savannah's mother, friended me on Facebook a year or so after Savannah's death but the connection lay dormant for a long time. But when, in November 2016, thousands of words flooded out of me and I realized that I had just begun writing a memoir, I knew the time had come for us to reconnect. I messaged Shannon and she responded right away, almost as if she had been waiting for a sign from me.

☞

We met at a quiet bistro in Hamilton's Westdale on a grey December afternoon. A small glass vase holding yellow, orange and white flowers brightened the table. I smiled at Shannon, nervous about how she would receive me, and perched on the chair opposite her.

"For you," Shannon said, twirling the vase. "Yellow was Savannah's favourite colour. And she loved butterflies." A sun-yellow tulle butterfly hovered on a large orange gerbera daisy.

Shannon talked about Savannah: her strength, her love of the ocean, the colour yellow and butterflies. Whenever she sees a butterfly, Shannon thinks that her daughter is there. She told me about Savannah meeting the country music superstar Reba McEntire backstage at her concert in Toronto and Reba's tears at Savannah's strength and determination. About Savannah's trip to Hawaii where she swam with dolphins in the turquoise sea. Shannon wanted to write about Savannah so that her daughter would continue to inspire people the way she had when she was alive.

"You absolutely should," I said and told her about a lovely writing studio on the Danforth in Toronto that supports people who were only starting to write.

Letting Shannon talk was good medicine – for both of us. I didn't need training in narrative medicine to realize that listening and attention were in order. It would have been inhuman to dump all my doubts and worries about Savannah onto Shannon. In the end, I did tell Shannon that I had been upset about Savannah for a long time and that I had thought that she had suffered in that tiny body of hers. But I also said that Shannon's unyielding and unending belief in Savannah and in her strengths taught me that Savannah had had a happy life, a wonderful and worthwhile life – a life I never expected for her when I saw her ultrasounds so long ago. That I had been wrong.

"I'm writing a memoir and Savannah's in it," I finished.

Shannon's eyes lit up.

☞

Two years later, in late January 2018, we met again for lunch in an empty bar, the only place open during a snowstorm that had battered Hamilton all morning. The weather had kept most of the lunchtime crowds away.

For over two hours we talked about Savannah's life. About her capacity for happiness. About my distress. I had never owned up to how miserable I felt – how responsible – every time I saw her in my clinic room. Shannon told me about her unshakable belief that Savannah continued to look over her and Shane and Jack: a five-dollar bill found on the sidewalk (five was Savannah's favourite number), a license plate with HI FIVE. She told me about Shane's chagrin after he'd read my narrative medicine article, which I had sent to Shannon after we first talked. It hurt him that I had not seen the wonder of Savannah and that I had put my feelings in print. We talked and talked. At one point, she asked what I had thought about her and Shane when we first met.

"You were the only person who supported us," she said. "And that's why it was so hard to feel you distance yourself after she was born."

So they had noticed – I wasn't as professional as I had hoped.

When I asked whether I could include Savannah's name and story in my memoir – and our story of reconnection – Shannon agreed without missing a beat.

"But you must ask Shane's permission, too," I said. "He had been so upset."

"He wants the world to know about Savannah," Shannon said. "How she changed the people she met." And she told me how the intensivist had said that Savannah made her believe in miracles, and how the neurosurgeon who operated on Savannah when she hit her head had written that Savannah had made her re-evaluate so many things she thought she knew. I sat there, remorseful that I only appreciated Savannah now, when it was too late; that I had to first wend my way through my misconceptions and prejudices before reaching that point. And that I had never experienced such unconditional acceptance. Shannon's love and pride in her imperfect daughter and the gifts Savannah had bestowed to the world shone through everything Shannon said.

☞

It was in writing about Savannah, in going back to her story and sharing it, that I realized that my entire life had been a quest for perfection, and that in my world, flaws – in myself as well as in others – were judged harshly, not tolerated. I began to question how I'd been brought up and taught, how the medical system had trained me to practice. All through my childhood, imperfection hadn't been tolerated, either in studying or in behaviour – harsh words and disapproval were meted out for every transgression. This produced a carapace, which I had spent years hiding underneath. And during my training, "being emotional" was frowned upon, the discouraging gazes of attendings and colleagues averted as if something shameful. But now, I learned that bottling up painful emotions because of shame led only to more misery. That it is better to acknowledge life's uncertainties than to pretend they do not exist. That doubts should be shared. I learned that people can be helpful, non-judgmental and accepting. That it is okay to be vulnerable.

Savannah gave me an amazing gift – my struggle, my misgivings about her life, have led me to recognize how important it is to share my pain. My task was to learn to be kind and forgiving toward myself. I didn't need to be perfect – good is good enough. Life is precious and fragile and wondrous and full of mistakes. Fail, fail better. Keep trying.

Acknowledgements

There were many people who helped me through the years of writing this memoir, and now comes the time to offer heartfelt thank yous:

- to Wolsak & Wynn Ltd. and to Noelle Allen, my careful and wise publisher, who have given this book a home;

- to Andrew Wilmot, for thoughtful comments and edits, and for eagle-eyed attention to all things spelling and punctuation;

- to Wayne Grady for his wisdom and for believing in this story well beyond what his job as a creative writing teacher and thesis advisor required;

- to Kasia Jaronczyk, my enabler in all things literary and writerly, and a dear, dear friend;

- to the genetic counsellors who make me look good every day;

- to Shannon and Shane Stanley for their heart and generosity in allowing me to share the story of their daughter, Savannah Rose;

- to the parents who allowed me to share their children's stories;

- to Jimm Douketis, for telling me that I am a writer before I believed it myself, for being my best friend, and for raising our two amazing sons with me – you not only are the rock upon which our lives are moored but you rock, too;

and, most importantly,

- to my patients and their families who teach me every day how precious and complicated life is and who imbue my work with meaning.

Thank you all.

Bibliography

Aase, Jon M. *Diagnostic Dysmorphology.* New York: Plenum Medical Book Company, 1990.

Behrman, Richard E., ed. *Nelson Textbook of Pediatrics.* 14th edition. Toronto: W.B. Saunders, 1992.

Bosk, Charles L. *All God's Mistakes.* Chicago: University of Chicago Press, 1992.

Braunwald, Eugene, Kurt J. Isselbacher, R.G. Petersdorf, Jean D. Wilson, Joseph B. Martin and Anthony S. Fauci, eds. *Harrison's Principles of Internal Medicine.* 11th edition. New York: McGraw-Hill Book Company, 1987.

Dillard, Annie. *For the Time Being.* New York: Alfred A. Knopf, 1999.

Ellis, Albert, and Raymond Chip Tafrate. *How to Control Your Anger before It Controls You.* New York: Citadel Press, 1997.

Farkas, Leslie G. *Anthropometry of the Head and Face.* 2nd edition. New York: Raven Press, 1994.

Goodwin, Frederick K., and Kay Redfield Jamison. *Manic-Depressive Illness.* New York: Oxford University Press, 1990.

Gorlin, Robert J., M. Michael Cohen and L. Stefan Levin. *Syndromes of the Head and Neck.* 3rd edition. New York: Oxford University Press, 1990.

Greene, Ross. *The Explosive Child: A New Approach for Understanding and Parenting Easily Frustrated, "Chronically Inflexible" Children.* New York: HarperCollins, 1998.

Hall, Judith G., Judith E. Allanson, Karen W. Gripp and Anne M. Slavotinek. *Handbook of Physical Measurements.* 2nd edition. New York: Oxford University Press, 2007.

Jones, Kenneth Lyons. *Smith's Recognizable Patterns of Human Malformation.* 4th edition. Toronto: W.B. Saunders, 1988.

Marion, Robert. *Genetic Rounds: A Doctor's Encounters in the Field that Revolutionized Medicine.* New York: Kaplan Publishing, 2010.

McKay, Matthew, Patrick Fanning, Kim Paleg and Dana Landis. *When Anger Hurts Your Kids*. Oakland, CA: New Harbinger Publications, 1996.

Phelan, Thomas W. *1-2-3 Magic: Effective Discipline for Children 2–12*. Glen Ellyn, IL: Child Management, Inc., 1995.

Rużyłło, Edward, ed. *Mała encyklopedia zdrowia*. 4th edition. Warsaw: Państwowe Wydawnictwo Naukowe, 1963.

Shem, Samuel. *The House of God*. New York: Richard Marek Publishers, 1978.

Stanisławski, Jan. *English–Polish/Polish–English Dictionary*. Warsaw: Państwowe Wydawnictwo: Wiedza Powszechna, 1979.

Wiedemann, Hans. *Atlas of Clinical Syndromes: A Visual Aid to Diagnosis for Clinicians and Practicing Physicians*. London: Wolfe Medical, 1985.